Effect of Yoga on M
Abil

L .Vijay

CONTENT

Sr. No.	Content	Page No.
	Content	i
	List of Table	iv
	List of Figure	vii
1.	**CHAPTER 1: INTRODUCTION**	1-31
	1.1 Yoga: Meaning of Yoga	5
	1.1.1 Need of Yoga Education	5-6
	1.1.2 Effect of Yoga Practices on Body and Mind	7
	1.2 Memory	7
	1.2.1 Memory in Terms of Types and Processes.	8
	1.2.2 Types of Memory	8-12
	1.2.3 The Memory Process	12-16
	1.2.4 Delayed Recall	16
	1.2.5 Remote Memory	17
	1.2.6 Attention	17
	1.2.7 Concentration	18
	1.2.8 How to Recall it	18-19
	1.3 Problem Solving Ability	19-20
	1.3.1 Problem-solving abilities were connected to a number of other skills, including	21-23
	1.3.2 The steps of problem solution were shown in the diagram below	23
	1.3.3 The Evaluation of problem consists of	24-25
	1.3.4 Problem solving ability and its role in sports performance:	25-26
	1.3.5 Yoga, psychology and problem solving ability	26-28
	1.4 Research Gap	28
	1.5 Statement of the Problem	28

	1.6 Objectives	28
	1.7 Hypothesis of the Study	28-29
	1.8 Delimitation of Study	29-30
	1.9 Limitations of Study	30
	1.10 Definition of the terms used	30-31
	1.11 Significance of the Study	31-32
2.	**CHAPTER 2: REVIEWS OF RELATED LITERATURE**	33-52
3.	**CHAPTER 3: METHOD AND PROCEDURE**	53-96
	3.1 Research Methods	53
	3.1.1 Design	53
	3.1.2 Sample and Training Programme	53-54
	3.1.3 Selection of Subjects	54
	3.1.4 Selection of Variables	55
	3.1.5 Criterion Measures	55
	3.1.6 Experimental Design	56
	3.2 Reliability of Data	56-57
	3.2.1 Validity	58
	3.3 Procedure for Data Collection	58-59
	3.3.1 Procedure for Administration of the Test	59-60
	3.3.2 Problem Solving Ability Test by L.N. Dubey (1971)	60-61
	3.4 Administration of Training Programme	61
	3.4.1 Contents of the training programme for each experimental group	61-96
	3.5 Statistical Techniques Used	96
4.	**CHAPTER 4: ANALYSIS AND INTERPRETATION OF DATA**	97-137
	4.1 Descriptive Statistics for Different Variables	97-108
	4.2 Effect of Yoga on Memory of Players from Different Universities	109-125
	4.3 Effect of Yogas on Problem Solving Ability of Players	126-134
	4.4 Correlation between memory and problem-solving ability	135-137

5.	**CHAPTER 5: RESULT, CONCLUSION AND RECOMMENDATIONS**	138-146
	5.1 Discussion of the Result	138-143
	5.2 Conclusion	143-145
	5.3 Recommendation for Further Studies	146
6.	**SUMMARY**	147-160

LIST OF TABLES

Table No.	Statement	Page No.
4.1.1	Descriptive statistics of PGI memory scale (PGI) and problem-solving ability test (PSAT) for pre and post of yoga camp for players from CDLU	97
4.1.2	Descriptive statistics of PGI memory scale (PGI) and problem-solving ability test (PSAT) for pre and post of yoga camp for players from CRSU	98
4.1.3	Descriptive statistics of PGI memory scale (PGI) and problem-solving ability test (PSAT) for pre and post of yoga camp for players from KUK	98
4.1.4	Descriptive statistics of PGI memory scale (PGI) and problem-solving ability test (PSAT) for pre and post of yoga camp for players from MDU	99
4.1.5	Descriptive statistics of subtests of PGI memory scale (PGI) before attending the yoga camp for players from CDLU	99
4.1.6	Descriptive statistics of subtests of PGI memory scale (PGI) after attending the yoga camp for players from CDLU	100
4.1.7	Descriptive statistics of subtests of PGI memory scale (PGI) before attending the yoga camp for players from CRSU	101
4.1.8	Descriptive statistics of subtests of PGI memory scale (PGI) after attending the yoga camp for players from CRSU	102
4.1.9	Descriptive statistics of subtests of PGI memory scale (PGI) before attending the yoga camp for players from KUK	103
4.1.10	Descriptive statistics of subtests of PGI memory scale (PGI) after attending the yoga camp for players from KUK	104
4.1.11	Descriptive statistics of subtests of PGI memory scale (PGI) before attending the yoga camp for players from MDU	105
4.1.12	Descriptive statistics of subtests of PGI memory scale (PGI) after attending the yoga camp for players from MDU	106
4.1.13	Descriptive statistics of subtests of PGI memory scale (PGI) before attending the yoga camp for all players	107
4.1.14	Descriptive statistics of subtests of PGI memory scale (PGI) after attending the yoga camp for all players	108

4.2.1	Difference in the results of the PGI memory scale test of the respondents before attending the yoga camp with respect to their universities	109
4.2.2	Comparison of the results of the PGI memory scale test of the respondents before attending the yoga camp with respect to their universities	110
4.2.3	Difference in the results of the PGI memory scale test of the respondents after attending the yoga camp with respect to their universities	111
4.2.4	Comparison of the results of the PGI memory scale test of the respondents after attending the yoga camp with respect to their universities	112
4.2.5	Difference in the gain in results of the PGI memory scale test of the respondents after attending the yoga camp with respect to their universities	113
4.2.6	Difference in the results of the PGI memory scale test of the respondents after attending the yoga camp with respect to their universities	114
4.2.7	Difference in the results of the remote memory test of the respondents after attending the yoga camp	115
4.2.8	Difference in the results of the recent memory test of the respondents after attending the yoga camp	116
4.2.9	Difference in the results of the mental balance test of the respondents after attending the yoga camp	117
4.2.10	Difference in the results of the attention and concentration test of the respondents after attending the yoga camp	118
4.2.11	Difference in the results of the delayed recall test of the respondents after attending the yoga camp	119
4.2.12	Difference in the results of the immediate recall test of the respondents after attending the yoga camp	120
4.2.13	Difference in the results of the retention for similar pairs test of the respondents after attending the yoga camp	121
4.2.14	Difference in the results of the retention for dissimilar pairs test of the respondents after attending the yoga camp	122

4.2.15	Difference in the results of the retention for dissimilar pairs test of the respondents after attending the yoga camp	123
4.2.16	Difference in the results of the recognition test of the respondents after attending the yoga camp	124
4.3.1	Difference in the results of the problem-solving ability test of the respondents before attending the yoga camp with respect to their universities	126
4.3.2	Comparison of the results of the problem-solving ability test of the respondents before attending the yoga camp with respect to their universities	127
4.3.3	Difference in the results of the problem-solving ability test of the respondents after attending the yoga camp with respect to their universities	128
4.3.4	Comparison of the results of the problem-solving ability test of the respondents after attending the yoga camp with respect to their universities	129
4.3.5	Difference in the gain in results of the problem-solving ability test of the respondents after attending the yoga camp with respect to their universities	130
4.3.6	Comparison of the gain in the results of the problem-solving ability test of the respondents after attending the yoga camp with respect to their universities	131
4.3.7	Difference in the results of the problem-solving ability test of the players after attending the yoga camp with respect to their universities	133
4.4.1	Correlation between results of the PGI memory scale test and problem-solving ability test of players from different universities of Haryana before attending the yoga camp	135
4.4.2	Correlation between results of the PGI memory scale test and problem-solving ability test of players from different universities of Haryana after attending the yoga camp	136

LIST OF FIGURES

Table No.	Statement	Page No.
4.2.1	University wise difference in the mean values of the results of PGI memory scale test for per and posy yoga camp	113
4.2.2	University wise gain in the PGI memory scale test results	114
4.2.3	Mean-wise difference in the performance of the remote memory test of the players, pre and post of attending yoga camp	116
4.2.4	Mean-wise difference in the performance of the recent memory test of the players, pre and post of attending yoga camp	117
4.2.5	Mean-wise difference in the performance of the mental balance test of the players, pre and post of attending yoga camp	118
4.2.6	Mean-wise difference in the performance of the attention and concentration test of the players, pre and post of attending yoga camp	119
4.2.7	Mean-wise difference in the performance of the delayed recall test of the players, pre and post of attending yoga camp	120
4.2.8	Mean-wise difference in the performance of the immediate recall test of the players, pre and post of attending yoga camp	121
4.2.9	Mean-wise difference in the performance of the retention for similar pairs test of the players, pre and post of attending yoga camp	122
4.2.10	Mean-wise difference in the performance of the retention for dissimilar pairs test of the players, pre and post of attending yoga camp	123
4.2.11	Mean-wise difference in the performance of the visual retention test of the players, pre and post of attending yoga camp	124
4.2.12	Mean-wise difference in the performance of the recognition test of the players, pre and post of attending yoga camp	125
4.2.13	Difference in the results of ten subtests of PGI memory scale test	125
4.3.1	University wise difference in the mean values of the results of problem-solving ability test for per and posy yoga camp	130
4.3.2	University wise gain in the problem-solving ability test results	132

CHAPTER 1
INTRODUCTION

Yoga is the oldest-known science of self-development, and has found to be the answer to modern machine age. There are many important heritages in India and yoga is one of them. It is one of the greatest gifts of India to the world. It manages the problems related with health, physical fitness and peace of mind. Yoga teaches us how to ameliorate and control the condition of every part of our body. Yoga and yogic practices have gained popularity all over the world. It has been one of the most popular systems of health and healing all over the world. Yoga is an ancient science, which has been practiced for more than millennia and is based on harmonizing systems of development for the body, mind and spirit, Kumar (2005). People in the past found it interesting how they lived and they composed their stories with letters. From one generation to another generation fundamental information is transferred in the form of fantasies. This is the method by which knowledge develops and becomes culture. Surely, yoga has been introduced in this way since the past. There is a lot of scope for improvement and development that can be achieved through yoga practice that is the treasure of our glorious land. Yoga today is not just a routine exercise but is a system that coordinates with science and has a positive effect on the body and mind. It has many benefits, for example pressure is reduced by yogic practices, it focuses on simplicity and softness, which is good for your mind and body. Now-a-days anxiety, mental tension and stress have become imminent companions of players. Yoga can reduce and cure illness as it creates the balance of positive and negative powers. The ultimate aim of Yoga is self-identification and self-perfection that comes through self-realization. It is a historic science and way of life, which include physical movements, pose, meditation and pranayama. Yoga practice can improve the players to focus on their mental resources, information processing more quickly and accurately and also learn to update information effectively.

Yoga can be used by everyone regardless of age, sex, physical condition, back ground etc. People use yoga to overcome their individual problems. Yoga can be used to correct the physical deformities of children and even elderly people. As we realize that the youngsters are the banks of energy and they are known as an equivalent of movement (dynamic). It is much harder to teach them yoga or static yogic asana.

Western countries are turning to yoga because it has been proved that yoga successfully counteracts the occupational pains that every person has these days. It is an art and science of healthy living acknowledged as the best means for wellness. There are innumerable benefits of yoga due to which the graph of yogic practices is raising quickly all throughout the planet. It is a way of life, which is beyond any religion, caste and country and can be practiced by the entire mankind.

Yogic practices are accepted to have tremendous mental and helpful qualities. Yoga has the surest solutions for men's mental health just as actual illnesses. For many people yoga is viewed as a physical, mental, and spiritual discipline that confers a sound body and a sound mind. Apparently, the practices of yoga can help a person achieve his or her full potential and helps increase spiritual consciousness. Breathing techniques and posture are two of the physical aims in yoga, while one of the mental aims is the ability to maintain cognitive control, specifically in the areas of attention, memory, and arousal control. One common claim is that yoga helps clear the mind and this may have an effect on the ability to attend to relevant stimuli and recall information subsequently, Heriza (2004).

For many Americans yoga became a very popular recreational activity. Relationship between the yogic practices and benefits related to mental health and overall wellness is apparent, Schaeffer (2002). Inverted yoga positions have been associated which claims to increase memory and attention due to increased blood flow to the brain. For example, Schaeffer (2002) claimed "yoga can prevent memory lapses by calming you and enhancing your concentration. It can also improve your powers to recall by increasing circulation to your brain".

Yoga aims at harmonizing the physical, mental and spiritual aspects of personality, with a view to attaining the highest level of consciousness. From the level of gross body to level of pure consciousness, yoga disciplines thus embraces the whole of the operational existence of human beings. This all embracing new awareness leads to correct understanding of one's own nature, which is a step towards gaining a total control over activities in all spheres and all the levels of one's existence. This is done through the practice of asana, pranayama, mudra, bandha, shatkarma and meditation, and must be achieved before union can take place with the higher reality, S.S. Saraswati (2009).

Yoga, the oldest Indian way of dealing with fitness is appreciated for considering the human being as the whole body, mind and spirit together and not in separate components. It helps the individual to connect with one's inner spirit, which is essentially divine and is connected to the 'universal spirit' or 'God'. Such an approach and philosophy is strongly anti-stress; disintegration of: his personality leads to stress. The aim of man's life is to get rid of the worries, anxieties and suffering of the world and to achieve peace.

The modern age is the age of stress, tension and anxiety, our environment is fighting for survival and we humans suffer from more and more physical and psychological stress, which we can't control but can learn how to face them and to this end yoga is as good an invention it has ever been. The main credit of systematizing yoga goes to Patanjali who wrote the" yoga sutra" two thousand years ago. He has recommended 8 stages of yoga discipline, yama (social code), niyama (personal code), asana (posture), pranayama (control of prana), pratyahara (sense withdrawal), dharana (concentration), Dhyana (meditation) and Samadhi (super consciousness), Awasthi (2015).

Yoga solves the problems of health, physical fitness and peace of mind. It is the science of right living and is intend to be incorporated in daily life. It works on all aspects of the person: the physical, vital, mental, emotional, psychic and spiritual. The science of yoga begins to work in the outermost aspect of the personality, the physical body, which for most people is a practical and familiar starting point. When imbalance is experienced at this level, the organs, muscles and nerves no longer function in harmony; rather they act in opposition to each other. For instance, the lymphatic, which is responsible for fighting infections and improving immunity, might work improperly. Due to yoga the continuous contraction and relaxation of muscles and movements of organs lymph drainage is facilitated which helps in maintaining a healthy lymphatic system. Yoga aims at bringing the different bodily functions into perfect coordination so that they work for the good of the whole body.

Fitness and Physical fitness - Both terms involve quality of life. Fitness includes emotional, mental, spiritual, social fitness and as well as physical fitness. Currently, a popular term for fitness is wellness. But terms fitness and physical fitness are often used interchangeably. Though, they do not mean the same, Miller, Davic K.(2006).

Yoga moves on to the mental and emotional levels from the physical body. Because of stresses and interactions of everyday life many people suffer from phobias and neuroses. Yoga can't provide a cure for life but it can help in coping up with these problems. By practicing yoga awareness develops on the interrelationship among the emotional, mental and physical levels, and how a disturbance in any one of these affects the others. Gradually, this awareness leads to an understanding of the more subtle areas of existence, S.S.Saraswati,(2009). The modern age is the age of stress, tension and anxiety. There are a number of ways in which yoga is beneficial for us for example it reduces tension, improves concentration, cleans respiratory organs, cures various diseases, keeps the correct posture and it also increases flexibility.

Now-a-days yoga is accepted as one of the best means for fitness. Yoga helps in reducing obesity, obese people fall prey to various diseases. By reducing mental tension through meditative asana obesity can also be reduced. The graph of yogic practices is rising rapidly around the globe. A number of surveys conclude that yogic practice gives a number of benefits spiritually, mentally and physically, Kauts,(2012).

On the basis of their nature of moments yoga can be classified into three types - Static yogic practices, dynamic yogic practices and Combination yogic practices. Yogic practices like Asana, Dharana, Dhyana which are static in nature fall under the category of Static yogic practices. Combination yogic practices (Suryanamaskar with slow pace and yogic asanas practice with slow rhythm and hold in the final pose of asana) are the combination of both Static and Dynamic practices. Combination yogic practices always give best results because it is involved in both anaerobic and aerobic metabolism of the body.

A healthy body results in a great physical as well as mental performance. Health is real wealth, not pieces of gold and silver but we often fail to understand that only a healthy body can look perfectly after and maintain good health for the family. In today's hectic lifestyle we need some extra care routine to follow for good health, Awasthi, (2015).

Now-a-days students are tired because of too much intellectual activity. They sit in overcrowded classrooms, cramped and bent over their books. Real education is for the inner understanding and the growth of a student in all fields. It is not just for the fulfillment of external, social and economic commitments by S.S.Saraswati, (2009). Yogic training programmes are very beneficial as they help in decreasing stress, anxiety and improve concentration and memory. Yogic practices are believed to have tremendous psychological and therapeutic values.

1.1 YOGA: MEANING OF YOGA

According to Swami Digamber ji "Yoga is a union of Atma and Paramatma". The term 'YOGA' is derived from the Sanskrit word 'YUJ'. The most acceptable meaning is "YUJ SAMADHU" which means integration, that is to put things in their proper order and perspective. From the technical point of view the terms "Samyamana" and "Samadhi" are more appropriate. Even though people tend to think that yoga is a series of exercises with twisted body poses, it is not so. Basically, it helps the individual to connect with one's inner spirit. As per Yogic scriptures the practice of Yoga leads to the union of individual consciousness with that of the Universal Consciousness, indicating a perfect harmony between the mind and body, Man & Nature. Yoga is a traditional and cultural science of India. Ayurveda includes yoga as a part of an ideal lifestyle and maintenance of health (swastha vritta). Hatha yoga, ashtanga yoga, bhakti yoga, mantra yoga, dhyana yoga, karma yoga, raj yoga appear like different types of yoga due to their different methods and techniques but the main objective of all of them is liberation, salivation or to attain Samadhi, the highest state of chitta (consciousness) by controlling its vrittis (tendencies, desires) arising in it, out of attachment with materialistic world, so as to merge into the divine principle (absolute consciousness). Yoga is an experiential science, M.M.Gore, (2012).

"Yoga" also refers to an inner science comprising of a variety of methods through which human beings can realize this union and achieve mastery over their destiny. Yoga, being widely considered as an 'immortal cultural outcome' of Indus Saraswati Valley civilization dating back to 2700 B.C., It has proved itself catering to both material and spiritual upliftment of humanity. The identity of Yoga Sadhana is the basic human values, Ishwar V.Basavaraddi, (2015).

1.1.1 Need of Yoga Education

Inner strength, good intellect along with physical nourishment to our body, is provided by yoga due to which people all over the world have taken to yoga practices.

Gradually the understanding of yoga is getting deepened. Various yogic practices such as surya namaskar, asana, pranayama and meditation were introduced along with the formal education in the ancient Indian systems of Education. Only bookish knowledge, examinations and job orientation have become the prime factors in the new education system and yoga practices like Surya Namaskar were forgotten. Majority of the students in our country are in a confused state of mind and have no idea of their future. At the primary level we have neglected the science of yoga. As we all know that yoga is the only technology, which can bring total personality development. But still little importance is given to physical education and sports, we still believe in classroom teaching. Moreover, most of the schools don't have playgrounds.

Promoting psychological wellness and dealing with psychological disorders is done by yoga. As some features and practices of yoga deals with such disorders and also promote psychological wellness. Yoga or yogic practices have many benefits, the first one is that it can induce harmony in mind-body functioning Singh A.P., Mishra G (2012). Second - As it is experientially-rooted; it can be adopted considerably with much ease in comparison to the existing psychological practices Kakar S (2003). Third, since training and taking the service of a yoga therapist is cost effective, it has promising potential to address mental health concerns of the people. In India, approximately $145 billion a month are saved which are spent to meet medication cost, doctor's fee, and travelling cost to meet the doctor and the credit for this goes to yoga as it helps in treatment of mental illness. There are indirect savings also which accrue owing to loss of wages, disability, absenteeism and unimaginable substance abuse. Fourth, Multiple physical, emotional and social sufferings can also be alleviated holistically. Efficiency of any psychological therapy is multiplied determined by factors either in the environment or in the attributes of the client or therapist but not by highly acclaimed theory-based techniques. The demand for personalized, eclectic, and intuitive therapeutic approaches is rising gradually. Consequently, use of yogic practices as an adjunct to other forms of psychotherapy, is frequently reported.

Yoga is also commonly understood as a therapy or exercise system for health and fitness. While physical and mental health is natural consequences of yoga, the goal of yoga is more far-reaching. "Yoga is about harmonizing oneself with the universe. It is the technology of aligning individual geometry with the cosmic, to achieve the highest level of perception and harmony." Ishwar V. Basavaraddi (2015).

1.1.2 Effect of Yoga Practices on Body and Mind:

Body and mind are positively affected by yoga asana. Continually practicing yoga helps to develop concentration of mind and spiritually connected with Supreme power. Practice of yoga asana has been followed from ancient times and will be followed continuously. These are best for the human system. They promote inner health and harmony by providing proper exercises and tone up every part of our body. Now a days students are going through assessment anxiety, absence of concentration. It is mandatory to do physical activities to protect oneself. The research scholar attempted to build a comprehensive extensive yoga training project to improve the status of the student's body just as psyche (mind) and soul.

1.2 MEMORY

Memory is the store of information learned and kept by an organism's activity or experience, as shown by structural or behavioral changes, as well as recall and recognition. It is the human brain's ability to encode, store, retain, and recall information and past experiences. The ability to recall or remember past events or previously learnt information or skills is called memory, Ellenbogen (2006).

Yogic training programs help in reducing pressure, tension and it improves concentration and memory. Dharna and Dhyana are beneficial for getting peace of mind and increasing concentration. Memory is the faculty of the brain by which data or information is encoded, stored and retrieved when needed. It is the retention of information over time for the purpose of influencing future action. If past events could not be remembered, it would be impossible for language, relationships, or personal identity to develop. Memory loss is usually described as forgetfulness or amnesia. Memory is often understood as an informational processing system with explicit and implicit functioning that is made up of a sensory processor, short-term memory and long-term memory. This can be related to neuron. The sensory processor allows information from the outside world to be sensed in the form of chemical and physical stimuli and attended to various levels of focus and intent. Working memory serves as an encoding and retrieval processor. Information in the form of stimuli is encoded in accordance with explicit to implicit functions by the working memory processor. The working memory also retrieves information from previously stored material, Patel (2019).

Memory is directly related to our brain; in fact it is the third eye of human beings. Though content can be acquired by the intelligent mind. Therefore, Yoga Asana was one of the most important methods to improve potential and solidity of learners.

Memory is a brain function that allows you to remember things. Where data is encoded, saved, and retrieved as required. Memory is crucial to experiences; it is the process of retaining information through time in order to influence future behaviour.

Memory is commonly thought of as an information processing system with explicit and implicit functions that consists of a sensory processor, a short-term (or working) memo, and a long-term (or permanent) memory.

Information from the outside world is sensed in the form of chemical and physical impulses, and varied levels of focus and intent are paid to by the sensory processor. Working memory is used for both encoding and retrieval. The working memory processor encodes information in the form of stimuli according to explicit or implicit functions. Information is also retrieved from previously stored data by the working memory. Long-term memory's job is to store information using various category models or systems.

1.2.1 Memory in Terms of Types and Processes

Types	1. Sensory Memory 2. Short -term Memory 3. Long -term Memory
Processes	1. Encoding 2. Storage 3. Retrieval

1.2.2 Types of Memory

1. Sensory memory

2. Short-term memory

3. Long-term memory

1) Sensory Memory

It enables us to retain sensory impressions after the original stimulus has stopped. Fast-moving lights in the dark are a common example. Echoic memory (the auditory sensory store) and haptic memory (the tactile sensory store) were the two types of sensory memory that have been investigated.

Visual information was stored in echoic memory for about a third of a second or longer. As an example,

Person #1.- "What time is it?"

Person #2.- "What did you say? "Oh, 2.30 ?"

After the first person asks the question, the second person hears it. This was due to echoic memory, which saves the second of the question for the second or two times it was asked. Even if you weren't paying attention when the words were spoken, you can hear them if you pay attention to them now, Patel (2019).

Sensory memory functions include preventing overwhelm, providing decision time, providing stability, playback, and recognition.

2) Short Term Memory

Working memory was another name for short-term memory. It only contains a few items (study indicates a range of 7 +/- 2 items) and only lasts around 20 seconds, implying that it only holds a limited quantity of data.

Short-term memory, on the other hand, can quickly transfer memories to long-term memory via rehearsal processes. When someone offers you a phone number over the phone, you repeat it to yourself until you can write it down.

Short-term memory functions include attending, which entails paying attention to relevant information while ignoring everything else, rehearsing, which entails holding information for a short period of time until you decide what to do, and storing, which entails storing or encoding information for the long term, Patel (2019).

a) Working Memory

Short-term memory and working memory were comparable. Working memory, on the other hand, was where a person manipulates information. Working Memory, consists of both verbal and visual components. They allow simultaneous processing of images and words on their way to storage, despite being different mental subsystems. Though one can communicate verbally while driving (visual processing), one cannot effectively engage in both verbal and visual dialogues at the same time since each of these subsystems has limitations, Baddeley (2002)

This aids them in remembering the specifics of their current assignment. Working memory was used in a variety of behaviours, including:

- o Solving a difficult arithmetic problem that requires multiple numbers to be remembered
- o Baking something that necessitates a person's memory of previously added ingredients
- o Taking part in a debate, in which one must recall the primary points and evidence presented by either side.

3) Long Term Memory

It was the system in our brain that stores, manages, and retrieves information. Long-term memory can be classified as procedural, primed, episodic, or semantic. Procedural memory was a type of implicit memory that allows people to accomplish actions without thinking about it; it was also known as "how to" information. The information was first stored in the motor cortex and then transferred to the cerebellum. Priming memory was an implicit memory that quickly biases the brain to non-conscious information. It was saved in the part of the cerebral cortex that processes the original stimuli.

Episodic memory was a declarative memory that recalls personal experiences through conscious thought. The hippocampus and the prefrontal cortex are both involved. Declarative memory, or semantic memory, was a type of declarative memory in which conscious thought summons previously learned information, such as facts about the world. It was possibly kept in the same area as episodic memory.

Everything from what we learned in first grade to our old addresses to what we wore to work yesterday was included in long-term memory. It has an enormous storage capacity, and some memories can remain from the moment they were formed until we die. (https://www.brainhq.com/brain-resources/memory/types-of-memory/)

Subcategories of long term memory are:

a) Explicit Memory

b) Implicit Memory

a) Explicit Memory: One of the two major subcategories of long-term memory was explicit memory (also known as "declarative memory"), and (Implicit memory was the other). Explicit memory necessitates conscious thought, such as remembering who came to supper last night or naming rainforest creatures. It's what most people think of when they hear the word "memory," whether it's a good or negative one. (https://www.verywellmind.com/implicit-and-explicit-memory-2795346)

Explicit memory was frequently associative; your brain connects memories. When you think of a phrase or an event, such as an automobile, your mind might conjure up a slew of recollections, ranging from carburetors to your commute to a family road trip and a thousand other things. (https://www.brainhq.com/brain-resources/memory/types-of-memory/explicit-memory/)

Explicit Memory works:

- Are stored in memory and retrieved later
- Rehearsals are frequently used to shape them.
- Unconsciously encoded and linked to emotions
- It's possible that associations will bring it to your attention.

Explicit Memory was divided into two parts:

i) Episodic Memory

ii) Semantic Memory

i) Episodic Memory: One sort of explicit memory was episodic memory. Episodic memory was autobiographical in that it serves as a vital record of our individual experiences. Our episodic memory permits us to recall details such as our trip to Vegas, what we ate for dinner the night before, and who informed us that our friend Maryann was pregnant. Any previous event in which we participated and which we recall as a "episode" (scene of events) was episodic. Several factors influence how effectively we remember an episodic memory.

ii) Semantic Memory: Semantic memory was another sort of explicit memory. It was responsible for our "textbook learning" and general world knowledge. It's what allows us to state things like "a zebra was a striped animal" or "Paris was the capital of France" without understanding when or where we learnt them. Scientists aren't sure where semantic memory takes place in the brain; some claim it happens in the hippocampus and adjacent locations, while others believe it happens all over. Semantic memory, like episodic memory, goes from strong (recall) to weak (remembering)(familiarity).(https://www.verywellmind.com/implicit-and-explicit-memory-2795346)

b) Implicit memory: Implicit memory stores information that people don't intend to recall. This type of remembering was both inadvertent and unconscious. Because you can't actively bring implicit memory into awareness, it's also referred to as non declarative memory.

Implicit memories those weren't aware and can't be expressed verbally. Implicit memories were frequently procedural in nature, focusing on the steps that must be followed to complete a task. https://www.brainhq.com/brain-resources/memory/types-of-memory/explicit-memory/

Implicit Memory works:

- With repetition, it becomes instinctive.
- Learning skills and mastering a task are the first steps.
- This can lead to priming, or the same response to similar stimuli.
- Is frequently reliant on context and cues.

Important memories were usually transferred from short-term to long-term memory. Information can be transferred to long-term memory in many stages for more permanent storage. Information can be committed to long-term memory by repetition, such as studying for a test or walking without thinking or by linking it with other previously learned knowledge, such as remembering a new acquaintance. Motivation was also a factor, because information about something you were passionate about more likely to be kept in your long-term memory.

That's why someone might remember a favorite cricket player's statistics or the store where a particular pair of shoes was purchased years after he retired, Zlonoga , B. (1986)

1.2.3 The Memory Process

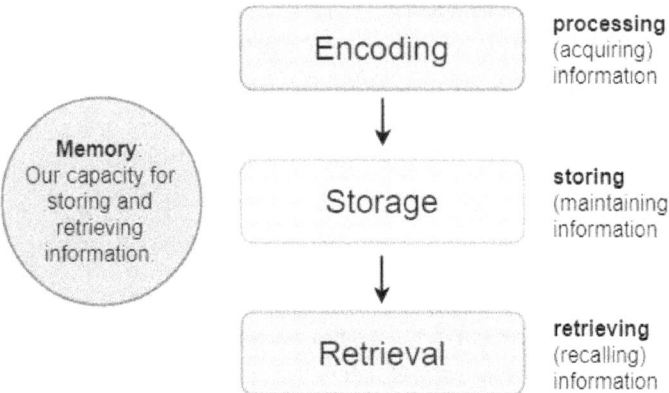

1). Encoding: Receiving, processing, and combining data was the process of encoding. Information from the outside world can enter our senses through encoding in the form of chemical and physical sensations.

2). Storage: The creation of a permanent encoded information record is referred to as storage. The second memory stage was storage, in which we keep information for long periods of time.

3). Retrieval or recall: The retrieval or recall of previously stored information in response to an event. This third stage was the recall of information that we have stored. We must find it and bring it back into our awareness. As a result of this information, some attempted retrievals may be simple, Patel (2019).

Encoding (mental processing of information so that it may be kept in memory), storage (keeping that information for a period of time), and retrieval were all part of the memory process (accessing or recalling stored memories when needed), Long-term memory (LTM) - items encoded into LTM are retained almost permanently; restricted in capacity (7 items) and duration (less than a minute unless actively practising), short-term memory (STM) – items encoded into STM are held virtually permanently; capacity that was nearly limitless Long-term memory (LTM) - things encoded into LTM are maintained almost permanently; practically infinite capacity (7 items) & duration (less than a minute unless actively rehearsing), long-term memory (LTM) - things encoded in LTM are stored indefinitely; nearly infinite capacity Sensory Memory stores the image for a short amount of time, providing continuity in our experience and allowing us to select whether or not to pay attention. Auditory sensory memory was referred to as echoic memory, Meltzoff, A. N., (1995).

Short-term memory permits you to recall information for a few seconds to a minute without having to rehearse it. It also has a very low capacity. Short-term memory was thought to rely mostly on an auditory code for retaining information, with a visual code playing a smaller role. Conrad discovered that test respondents had more difficulty recalling acoustically identical groupings of letters (e.g. E, P, D). When people have trouble remembering acoustically similar letters instead than visually similar letters, it means the characters were encoded acoustically. Work, on the other hand, is concerned with the encoding of written text, thus while acoustic components may play a role in written language memory, generalizations to all types of memory are not possible, Conrad's, (1964).

Sensory memory and short-term memory storage capacity and endurance are generally restricted, implying that information was not maintained permanently. Long-term memory, on the other hand, can store significantly bigger amounts of data for possibly indefinite periods of time (sometimes a whole life span). It has an enormous storage capacity. For example, we may recall a random seven-digit number for only a few seconds before forgetting it, indicating that it was stored in our short-term memory. On the other hand, with repetition, humans can retain telephone numbers for many years; this knowledge was referred to as long-term memory. Long-term memory encodes information semantically, but short-term memory encodes it acoustically: It was discovered that after 20 minutes, test subjects had the most trouble recalling a group of words with similar meanings (e.g. big, large, grate) Episodic memory, which "attempts to capture information such as 'what,' 'when,' and 'where,'" was another aspect of long-term memory. Individuals who have episodic memory can recall specific events like birthday celebrations and weddings.

For being a good student it is important to have a good memory as it helps him to learn fast as well as to reproduce when required. Due to poor memory capacity most of the students fail to achieve their targets and goals. Memories have a major role in one's day to day life. One has to remember the things he has to do, he has to remember the telephone numbers, day to day account numbers and even bus numbers and so on. Children have to read and learn a lot according to their syllabus and routine.

Yogic training programs help in reducing pressure, tension and it improves concentration and memory. Dharna and Dhyana are beneficial for getting peace of mind and increasing concentration.

Evocative is connected to but distinct from learning, in this process we acquire knowledge of the surrounding and change our subsequent behaviour. While learning skills our neurons that release together to generate a specific experience are different, thus they have the ability to fire together again. To set an example we learn new things as a language by the help of outer resources but during its application we use our memory rather than books or outer resources. Therefore memory depends on one's learning skills, which represent how we store and retain learning information. But learning also depends on some limitations on memory.

Memory is stored by our mind, which provides the structure to new knowledge which is linked by association. This performance of human beings to call and learn their past memories in order to visualize upcoming time plans is a hugely advantageous attribute in our survival and development as a species, Ellenbogen, (2006).

Memory is the ability of the human brain to encode, store, retain, and recall information and prior events. The process of imprinting a memory starts the moment we are born and continues throughout our lives. For instance, we learn how to tie our shoes. Once we've mastered the procedure, it's stored in our long-term memory, and we can carry it out without having to think about the stages, Cornad,R.,(1964).

Sensory Memory stores the image for a short length of time, providing continuity in our experience and allowing us to select whether or not to pay attention, as well as iconic memory – visual sensory memory, auditory memory – echoic memory.

Yoga helps in developing good thinking, providing good exercise and it also helps in developing good discipline, preparing the children for enhancing their memory. Yogic knowledge and practices are the reason behind the good memory of Saints and sages of our country. Moreover, yoga exercises help the brain cells to receive more blood and help in the optimal level of functioning which results in good memory. Good thinking and good discipline are developed by observing 'Yama' and 'Niyama' (the Universal commandments and personal Disciplines).

Yogic exercises have an immediate effect on the mind of a person. For testing immediate (short-term) verbal memory abilities of college-aged males and females according to Kocher (1974) used both yogic exercises and nonsense syllables. The results which were recorded after a period of one-month yoga training for college-aged males and females suggested that yoga did facilitate immediate memory performance as compared in absence of yoga, and the benefit was greater for males than for females. According to Crooks (1991) the word 'Memory' has a dual meaning. It refers to a process or process by which we store and store information that we just need to remember later.

Manjunath and Telles (2004) compared the performance scores of two groups aged 11 to 16 on verbal and spatial memory. From the two groups's one attended yoga camp and the other a fine arts camp. The results were recorded after 10 days of their respective interventions. The yoga group showed a significant increase (43%) in spatial memory while the fine arts (and a control group) showed no change. Anantharaman and Kabir (1984) reported that memory span and attention was increased after the yoga training .The Indian legacy, yoga has also been utilized with limited positive results in rehabilitation with mentally retarded individuals and in training visual perceptual sensitivity, Manjunath & Telles, (2000).

A similar test was done by Sahasi (1989). But this time the effects of yoga were observed on five cognitive tests (color cancellation, digit forward, digit backward, recognition, and visual retention). The time span of the test was an academic year and the participants were 12 year old. From the beginning to the end of the school year both the groups showed improvement. However, the statistical analysis provided did not directly compare the control and experimental groups, stating only that the mean score of the experimental group was "slightly higher" than that of the controls.

1.2.4 Delayed Recall

The ability to recall specific knowledge after a time of rest or distraction from that information is known as delayed recall. This is sometimes used to assess memory skills in intelligence/aptitude tests. (https://www.alleydog.com/glossary/definition-cit.php?term=Delayed+Recall)

It is one of the tests that we use to diagnose Alzheimer's disease. In this test, some material is given to the person for remembering, the material is either a list of words or a paragraph and later on that person is asked to recall those words. Significant improvement was shown by yoga group in immediate and delayed recall of verbal

(RAVLT), visual memory (CFT), attention and working memory (WMS-spatial span), verbal fluency (COWA), executive function (Stroop interference) and processing speed (Trail Making Test-A) as compared to waitlist group.

1.2.5 Remote Memory

The ability of a person to remember things and events for many years is called remote memory. This is a function of long-term memory, which the brain stores differently than recent or short-term memories. Short-term memories are stored in different areas of the brain than long-term memories. (https://www.alleydog.com/glossary/definition .php?term=Remote+Memory)

1.2.6 Attention

The mental function that makes an individual fully conscious of an element in the environment is called attention. It may be a tool that block out stimuli that are not immediately relevant. Paying attention is the first step in the learning process. The role of attention in one's life starts from the stage of infancy. From approximately 3 months to 12 months of age infants pay attention towards the things that seem surprising or discrepant from what they know. The ability to be attentive increases with the age for auditory as well as for visual input. When a child grows older and older his ideas become stronger and clearer. He learns to select the stimuli he likes. He can focus his attention to get his desirable outcome. He also pays more attention to things, which interest him, more. As a component of learning, attention plays a vital role in the learning process. A task was completed successfully when it is done without any distraction. The deviated mind affects the attention process for lack of concentration. Both concentration and attention were interrelated. Weak concentration leads to poor attention. By using the determinants of attention such as size, colour, Intensity, position, directionality, and movement, and novelty etc., attention can be improved.

The ability to focus on auditory as well as visual input can be increased by the determinants of attention. Mind should be calm and receptive before paying attention to anything because a restless person can't pay attention to anything. Through the practice of yoga, this calm mind can be achieved. Yoga not only strengthens the body but also prepares the mind for the learning process. One with a sound body and sound mind achieves better in life. Optimum level of attention was possible only with a healthy and sound mind. Children develop attention with the practice of yoga, which prepares both body and mind.

1.2.7 Concentration

Concentration was a term used in everyday language, which means the ability to give all your attention or effort to something. Interviews with high-profile athletes revealed that lack of concentration was the main reason for poor performance. Not surprisingly therefore, concentration was a concept the layperson feels that they understand immediately. To improve concentration skills one should know what to concentrate on and should focus attention on those factors as improving concentration skills was not simply a case of trying harder to concentrate. Concentration was the process by which all thoughts and senses are focused totally upon a specific object or activity to the exclusion of everything else, which changes over time and maintaining the intensity, and focus of concentration requires effort. Recognizing this factor was important because it means that concentration can vary in both intensity and focus.

We can be focusing on the key parts of performance at one moment, but be distracted the next. Racket sport requires high-level concentration. Concentration or selective attention was also involved in racket sports because it was a psychological factor such as fatigue, state of situation, balance and functioning of the central nervous system which was important at time of playing the shots in different sports, Routledge and Paul Kegan (2004).

1.2.8 How to Recall it

- Remember something else: If you're having trouble remembering anything, think of something else that was linked to it. Remember the example the instructor used during the lecture if you can't recall specific facts. Brainstorming was a great way to refresh your memories. When you were stuck on a test, start putting down a bunch of related problem answers. It was very likely that you'll get the answer you're looking for.

- Pay attention to the commemoration: Observe the easily recalled facts and inquire of oneself to discover one's own natural memory processes. If one notices that he or she was having trouble remembering knowledge, one can alter or change the remembering/learning approaches to accommodate this.

- Use it before you forget it: If you want to remember something, read it, write it, say it, listen to it, and apply it as much as possible. Use a variety of methods to stay in touch with the content on a frequent basis. Studies groups were particularly useful since they allow you to teach the content to other students while also allowing you to focus your attention.

- Keep in mind that you never forget: Adopt an attitude that says, "I always remember everything, and if I have any trouble recalling any minor thing within my memory, I only have to find it," and this optimistic thinking actually works!

1.3 PROBLEM SOLVING ABILITY

In today's life we were facing lots of problems. Our problem solving ability helps us to solve it productively. It helps us to understand the matter clearly and react accordingly. It was an essential part for Physical activity and plays a vital role. Go across it and demonstrate them sharp sighted. It was all about using logic and imagination. Coherence the situation and come up with valuable results. Problem solvers actively anticipate potential future problems and act to prevent them or to mitigate their effects. A problem was a task for which a person has no easily available procedure for solving it, Dostal (2015). With advancements in socioeconomic and technological domains, an individual's life was becoming increasingly complicated, with a growing number of challenges. Problem solving abilities refers to the process of overcoming challenges or problems that obstruct the fulfillment of desires.

Problem-solving skill varies in kind and process from person to person. It fluctuates depending on the severity of the problem and the learners' abilities. Animals address problems by habitual behaviour or the trial-and-error method. Animals at a higher evolutionary level use insight to address their issues. The most significant way of problem solving in humans was reasoning", Gupta,(2013).

Cognition was a mental function that involves gathering information and processing it for purposes such as thinking, problem solving, and so on. In sports, cognitive talents were essential to make quick and effective decisions, select the appropriate tactics at the appropriate time, and anticipate respectively, of movement. Perceptual and psychomotor abilities are included in cognitive ability.

Higher order functions include working memory, reasoning, and cognitive flexibility. In order to solve a problem, all of these elements must be present. Gould and Logue,(2014) integrated problem-solving capacity as part of the human brain's executive function.

We experience issues in every aspect of life and attempt to overcome them using various means and approaches. As a result, having effective problem-solving skills was required to deal with challenges in many aspects of life. There were a wide range of difficulties that might arise in daily life, and anyone can be affected by them.

Problem solving is a method of meeting the needs of an unknown situation by applying previously acquired knowledge, insight, and competence. Problem solving skill was the ability to learn new techniques, tactics, and plans to overcome obstacles and solve difficulties in order to reach a goal, Thornton, (1998). Improving students' problem-solving abilities was one of educational psychology's biggest difficulties, and it's a big ask for any educational institution, Mayer and Wittrock, (2006).

With this in mind, it's no surprise that problem solving has recently been acknowledged as a fundamental domain that supports traditional literacy concepts in high school topics by educational large-scale assessments (LSAs) around the world. Problem solving was a method of overcoming obstacles that appear to be impeding the achievement of a goal." Regardless of inference, it was also a method of making adjustments, Gupta & Kavita, (2015).

According to D'Zurilla et al., (2007), self-confident people have a greater magnitude of problem-solving talents, giving them the belief that they can solve any problem. Problem solving, according to Farayola and Senduran, (2015), is a complicated mental process that entails envisioning, imagining, manipulating, analysing, abstracting, and associating ideas. They went on to say that issue solving is a process that starts with the first interaction with the problem and continues with the solution being evaluated in light of the available data. Problem solving can be characterised as a goal-directed sequence of cognitive, emotive, and cognitive actions focused toward finding an unknown entity for bridging a gap between a present and a desired state, based on all of the aforementioned definitions.

Problem solving was a mental process that involves identifying, analyzing, and resolving a problem. The main goal of issue solving was to remove any barriers or conditions that prevent you from achieving your intended outcome or goals.

Identification of a problem, definition of an issue, gathering information about a problematic situation, allocating resources to fix the problem, and tracking progress were all part of problem resolution.

1.3.1 Problem-Solving Abilities were Connected to a Number of other Skills, Including

- Analytical skills
- Innovative and creative thinking
- A lateral mindset
- Adaptability and flexibility
- Level-headedness
- Initiative
- Resilience (in order to reassess when your first idea doesn't work)
- Team working (if problem solving was a team effort)
- Influencing skills (to get colleagues, clients and bosses to adopt your solutions).

Recognize the problem for upcoming ideas and use it for solving essential elements of business. It was a weapon to use for good direction. Problem solving consists of using extempore to find out solutions in sequencing manner. Some of the problem-solving techniques developed and used in philosophy, artificial intelligence, computer science, engineering, mathematics, medicine and societies in general were related to mental problem-solving techniques studied in psychology and cognitive sciences.

Depending on the discipline, the term "problem solving" has a slightly varied connotation. In psychology, it was a mental process, while in computer science, it was a computerized process. There are two categories of problems: ill defined and well-defined, and each requires a distinct strategy. Issues that were well defined have distinct end goals and clearly expected solutions, whereas problems that are ill-defined do not. In comparison to ill-defined difficulties, well-defined problems allow for more initial planning. When it comes to solving difficulties, it's sometimes necessary to consider pragmatics, or how context influences meaning, as well as semantics, or how the problem was interpreted. The ability to comprehend the problem's final purpose and the rules that could be used to solve it was crucial to its resolution. Sometimes an issue necessitates abstract thinking or the development of a novel solution.

One of the trademarks of human intellect was the ability to tackle complex issues, MacLellan, Langley, & Walker (2012). Problem solving encourages youngsters to "consider themselves and others, as well as to acquire knowledge of self in the context of society."

It's a method of arriving at a solution that involves more than just using a previously acquired approach. A student with effective problem solving ability can be defined by their use of a variety of problem-solving tactics, solid arithmetic abilities, high self-confidence, checking responses for reasonableness, and capacity to analyze and solve the problem using critical and analytical skills.

According to Henderson et al (1953), issue solving requires a goal, individual blocking of that objective, and individual acceptance of that goal. Problem solving, according to Ausubel (1968), was a type of discovery learning that bridges the gap between a learner's prior knowledge and a solution to a problem. Here, issue solving will rely primarily on the learner's prior/existing knowledge, which must be applied to the circumstance at hand. However, measuring or keying into previous knowledge was not always simple, as it is dependent on a variety of factors.

Problem Solving, is a goal-directed cognitive learning process that employs previously learned knowledge and cognitive methods. This perspective on problem solving sees it as a learning process involving cognitive controls like cognitive style and meta-cognition, as well as relying on prior information. Padgette (1991) also noted that problem solving is an art that entails knowing all the rules—all of them, not just the point–by–number type—and then knowing which ones to break in any particular situation. As a result, any problem situation has three key characteristics: the provided, the aim, and the obstacles. The constituents, their relationships, and the criteria are presented.

"Modeling the problem and generating and confirming hypotheses by gathering and evaluating data, utilizing pattern analysis, graphing, or computers and calculators," according to Lajoie (1992). This definition emphasizes on the formulation, inquiry, and verification phases, but it leaves out the crucial aspects of Polya's looking back phase.

Problem-solving ability or skills, according to Goldstein and Levin (1987), was a complicated process that encompasses higher-order intellectual and cognitive processes. Blanchard-Fields (2007) distinguished between two sorts of problems: those with a single solution and those with several solutions.

An issue occurs when an individual fails to fulfill particular aims, which may be due to a barrier. Frustration arises when one encounters an impediment in achieving one's objectives.

Environmental stressors can be effectively managed with the support of society, friends, or one's own self. Problem solving may be learned, and it improves with practice and right instruction.

According to Gulsen (2008), certain specific challenges demand cognitive, tactical, and psychosocial talents, but most problems may be solved with simple thinking. Part of complex decision making was problem-solving procedure in a very hopeless situation or incoherent circumstances. Individual problem-solving capacity was required for complex decision-making. In other words, problem-solving skill was linked to problem-solving ability.

Evaluation, identification, selection of the best solution, and review of the action taken were all steps of problem solving.

1.3.2 The Steps of Problem Solution were shown in the Diagram below

Evaluation the problem
Gather information
Identify solution
Break problem into parts
Select best solution
Take action
Test and review
Examine results

1.3.3 The Evaluation of Problem Consists of

1. Clarification of the nature and magnitude of the problem was required for problem evaluation.
2. Statement of problem in negative form
3. Gathering data on the issue
4. Effectively organizing data or information.
5. Condensing the information that is available.
6. Making a decision on the problem-solving objectives.

The management of an issue was the second stage of problem solving:

1. Use of information gathered in a meaningful way and in a timely manner.
2. To analyze a problematic situation, divide or break it down into small segments so that it can be managed effectively.
3. A thorough examination of the various options for resolving the issue.
4. Actions that can be taken to achieve the goals.

Making decisions was the third level of issue solving. This stage consists of the following elements:

1. To make a decision about the options available for a specific set of actions.
2. Is more information required before making a decision or taking action to solve the problem?
3. To assess resources for solving a specific problem, decision-making is required.

The fourth stage was to solve the problem, with the final step being to monitor the outcome.

Problem solving skill refers to the process of overcoming challenges or problems that obstruct the fulfillment of desires. Problem solving differs in nature and technique from person to person.

Problem solving was a mental activity that is part of a bigger problem-solving process that also involves problem identification and problem structuring. Problem solving has been defined as a higher-order cognitive process that requires the modulation and control of more routine or fundamental skills. It was considered the most complex of all intellectual functions. When an organism or artificial intelligence system has to go from a given state to a desired goal state, problem solving was required. Problem-solving activities engage students in the learning process and encourage them to apply higher-order thinking skills. The application of principles and facts to explain novel events or forecast outcomes from known situations was referred to as problem solving. To build cause and affect relationships in physical phenomena, problem solving necessitates prediction, analysis of data, and principles. In general, our everyday activities were routine, and we have little difficulty carrying out our daily responsibilities. However, this was not always the case; occasionally, we were confronted with a difficult situation that works as a roadblock to achieving our objectives. These barriers might be physical, social, or economic, and they can stymie an individual's progress toward their goals.

As an alternative to exams and diagnostic categories for identifying pupils who require special services, problem solving can be used Andrea Carta,(2004). Problem solving refers to the framework or pattern that allows for innovative thinking and reasoning. It's the ability to reason and think at different levels of complexity. Unsatisfied desires and drives produce a condition of tension that allows the individual to put out his best effort and use his finest linguistic techniques, observations, forecasts, and interferences to overcome the obstacles that obstruct his progress toward his wants and fulfillment goals.

1.3.4 Problem Solving Ability and its Role in Sports Performance

The relationship between cognition and sports performance is multiplex. This helps to make quick decisions in any complex field. Moreover, Sports positive for countless problem to solve, with decision generally falling into two categories: systematic and spontaneous young athletes make systematic decision when they have some time to work with and can give deeper thoughts to situation and problem like the effort needed to decide whether to play on a travel sports team, or to try and play sports during the some sports seasons. When figuring out these questions, kites learn how to brainstorm multiple solutions, how to weigh options, how to seek mentoring and support, and how to commit to a final decision. These kinds of problem solving skills were positive for countless applications beyond sports and prepare kites with a skill set they will use for the rest of their lives. In addition, spontaneous decisions were also very important and include whether there is not much time to think and process.

For instance: spontaneous decision making include adjusting in game challenges quickly bouncing back from adversity, pulling teammates together during tough stretches, and working through bumps and bruises that occur during a game with spontaneous decisions, there is not much time to think through problems, promoting sportspeople too quickly. Find solutions and implement their ideas almost immediately. General executive function in the form of problem-solving skills, according to Agashe and Shambharkar (2014), is vital in sporting success. Executive functions such as problem-solving skills make up the global cognitive control. A good sportsperson's characteristic is the ability to solve challenges both on and off the field (Volkamer, 2009). Issue-solving ability may fall under the category of psycho-cognition, which involves making quick decisions in order to solve a problem.

Hristovski (2012) also shared a factor that increased sports performance. Likewise, Problem solving ability was proved to be very adventurous for those people who were involved in sports activities. As per theory of Newell Shaw and Simon (1958) sports persons tackle many problems in playgrounds. However, reducing problems such as competitive opponents creates many situations that are distracting and difficult to reach. So those men who have this creative ability play on a national level with full of efficiency and confidence. The global cognitive control reported that problem-solving ability practice future steps of an upon it by using mental ability.

1.3.5 Yoga, Psychology and Problem Solving Ability

Psychology: problem solving in psychology refers to the process of finding solutions to problems encountered in life. An individual's psychological adaption, self-confidence, communication efficiency, decision-making style, academic and social self-esteem were all intimately tied to issue solving." Problem resolution was linked to an individual's psychological adaption, self-confidence, communication efficiency, decision-making style, academic and social self-esteem (Korkut, 2002).

Most of the time, the solutions to these issues are circumstance or context specific. The problem was discovered and simplified in the first step of the process, which was problem discovery and problem shaping. The next step is to generate and evaluate potential solutions. Finally, a solution was chosen, which will be implemented and tested. Problems have a destination, and how you get there was determined by problem orientation (problem-solving coping style and skills) and methodical analysis. Introspection, behaviourism, simulation, computer modelling, and experiment were some of the tools used by mental health practitioners to explore human problem-solving processes. Social psychologists investigate the problem's person- environment interaction as well as problem-solving approaches that were independent and interconnected. Problem solving was a higher-order cognitive activity and intellectual function that necessitates the modulation and control of more fundamental or everyday talents, Bryson, M. (1991)

Numerous tactics and elements influence everyday issue solving, according to empirical study, Buchner, A. (1995). Deficits in emotional control and reasoning can be remediated with effective rehabilitation, according to rehabilitation psychologists studying people with frontal lobe injuries. This could improve injured people's ability to solve everyday problems Dorner, D (1975).

There are a number of studies, which shows that yogic practices have a positive effect on Memory and Problem Solving Abilities. Several yogic studies have shown improvement in memory and problem solving ability. Studies have shown that Yoga asanas, pranayama and meditation help in enhancing memory and improving attention. Chanting group has shown better results as compared to non-chanting practitioners. Chanting group showed significant increased scores in both the memory tests and considerable reduction in total error and total time taken for cancellation tests compared to non-chanting practitioners, Ghaligi (2006).

The aim of the research was to determine the effect of problem solving training on decision-making skill and critical thinking in emergency medical personnel. The results revealed that decision-making and critical thinking score in emergency medical personnel are low and problem solving course' positively affected the personnel' decision making skill and critical thinking after the education programme, Heidari, (2016).

It has been proven by the research that regular practice of yoga helps in the development of the body, mind, and spirit, leading to healthier and more fulfilling life, Ray, et al, (2001). Apart from achieving physical health, yoga can maintain cognitive control, specifically in the area of attention and memory, Heriza, 2004; Oken et al, (2006). Various studies and surveys have been conducted to analyze the effect of yoga practices on attention, concentration and memory, Anantharaman & Kabir, (1984). The results showed that yoga shows a positive impact on mental health and wellbeing, attention –concentration, memory and physical fitness. Yoga have many benefits in a student's life as it can increase a student's ability to concentrate, focus and improve memory, Galanpino et al, (2008). Incorporating physical activity into daily lives of students is essential to their health and well-being, Williams & Ellis, (2013). Yoga is the form of physical activity entering schools, which increases academic performance and stimulates the brain Harr, Doneyko and Lee, (2012).

1.4 RESEARCH GAP

The present study focused upon the effect of Yoga practices on Memory and Problem Solving Abilities of the University yoga players. There are various researches done in past which shows the impact of Yoga on Memory of the players. However, there are lacunae of literature which demonstrated the effect of Yoga on Problem Solving Abilities. Moreover, the correlation between the Memory and Problem Solving Abilities was also seen in the present study which was not shown in the previous studies. The present study is an attempt to explore the effect of Yoga on Memory and Problem Solving Abilities of University Yoga players.

1.5 STATEMENT OF THE PROBLEM

The purpose of the study was to see the **"Effect of Yoga on Memory and Problem Solving Ability of Players"**.

1.6 OBJECTIVES

The present study asserts to meet the following objectives:

1.) To find out the effect of the Yoga on Memory of Players.
2.) To find out the effect of the Yoga on Problem Solving Ability of Players.
3.) To find out the correlation between Memory and Problem Solving Ability of Players.

1.7 HYPOTHESIS OF THE STUDY

On the basis of the knowledge reflected by the available literature, research finding, experts opinion and the scholars own understanding of the problem it was hypothesized that:

1-There will be no significant difference of Yoga on Memory of Players.

- 1. a). There will be no significant difference of Yoga on Remote Memory of Players.
- 1. b). There will be no significant difference of Yoga on Recent Memory of Players.
- 1. c). There will be no significant difference of Yoga on Mental Balance of Players.
- 1. d). There will be no significant difference of Yoga on Attention and Concentration of Players.
- 1. e). There will be no significant difference of Yoga on Delayed Recall of Players.
- 1. f). There will be no significant difference of Yoga on Immediate Recall of Players.
- 1. g). There will be no significant difference of Yoga on Retention for Similar Pairs of Players.
- 1. h). There will be no significant difference of Yoga on Retention for Dissimilar pairs of Players.
- 1. i). There will be no significant difference of Yoga on Visual Retention of Players.
- 1. j). There will be no significant difference of Yoga on Recognition of Players.

2-There will be no significant difference of Yoga on Problem Solving Ability of Players.

3-There will be no significant Correlation between Memory and Problem Solving Ability of Players.

1.8 DELIMITATION OF STUDY

Keeping in view the limitations of time and other resources available, the present study was confined to the following delimitation:

- Related research work was delimited to the players of Universities of Haryana (Chaudhary Devi lal University, Sirsa; Chaudhary Ranbir Singh University,

Jind; Kurukshetra University, Kurukshetra; Maharishi Dayanand University, Rohtak).

- Related research work was delimited to psychological test PGI Memory Scale developed by Dwarka Pershad (1977) and Problem Solving Ability Test developed by L.N. Dubey (1971).
- Related research work was delimited to the age group between 20 to 25 years only.
- The research work was delimited to the 100 players (25 from each university).
- The research work was delimited to Yoga i.e. Asans, Pranayama, Kriya, Surya Namaskar.
- Related research work was delimited to the find out the effect of yogas on Memory (Remote Memory, Recent Memory, Mental Balance, Attention and Concentration, Delayed Recall, Immediate Recall, Retention for Similar pairs, Retention for Dissimilar Pairs, Visual Retention and recognition) and Problem Solving Ability of Players.

1.9 LIMITATIONS OF STUDY

The present study was the following limitation:

- All the players of the present study belong to Haryana.
- It was beyond control of the lifestyle and daily routine of players.
- The tool for collecting data was based on a psychological questionnaire.
- The data was based on the thoughts of the responders, which will not be completely free from these individual biases and prejudice.

1.10 DEFINITIONS OF THE TERMS USED

Yoga: According to Yoga Sutras: Yoga is the removal of the fluctuations of the mind.

According to Oxford (1990): Yoga - Hindu system of philosophic Meditation and asceticism designed to reunion with the universal spirit.

Memory: **According to Dr J. Z. Patel:** Memory consists in remembering what has previously been learnt.

Problem Solving Ability: According to Thomas J. D'Zurilla (1995): Problem Solving as a "cognitive–affective–behavioral process through which an individual (or group) attempts to identify, discover, or invent effective means of coping with problems encountered in everyday living".

Asana: According to Joshi (1960): The Static condition and posture of the body, delightfully was called asana.

Pranayam: According to Swami Kuvalayendra (1993): Pranayam to get control over the taking and releasing breath according to desire is called.

1.11 SIGNIFICANCE OF THE STUDY

Being the tallest, fastest, or strongest athlete in the world is great, but if a sportsperson lacks mental/cognitive skills, his or her entire performance will suffer. In the past, studies compared the psychological traits of players. Surprisingly, athletes psychological capacity has not been evaluated from a cross-cultural perspective.

In this regard, memory and problem-solving ability were evaluated in the current study since these two variables contain a wide range of psychological and cognitive elements. As a result, the findings of the proposed study will shed light on differences in memory and problem-solving ability among Haryana players, allowing sports psychologists to develop even more effective psycho- cognitive programmes for players while taking into account the impact of cultural diversity on these two variables.

- The study may be helpful to improve the physical and psychological status of individual.
- This study would promote awareness of physical activity and yoga among students, parents and teachers.
- The results of the study may highlight that if yoga training is effective for the selected variables.
- It would provide guidance and new knowledge to the physical education and yoga teachers.
- It shall promote children interest in yogasana.

- The study shall be torch bearer for the future investigators who were interested to find out the prevailing situation in children mental abilities and problem solving abilities.
- Maintaining a good mental health is crucial to live a long healthy life. Good mental health can enhance sportsmanship quality of life, while poor mental health can prevent players from living and enhancing life.

CHAPTER 2
REVIEW OF RELATED LITERATURE

In the presented chapter, the researcher presented research journals, dissertations, books, thesis reviews and other information sources. The investigation is related to the problem which is one of the most important steps towards any research study plan.

A review of the related literature provides a broad view of the subject, its relevance, importance, and practicality of the subject. The researcher needs to get updated information about what has been done in the particular field from which he wants to take a problem for research. A review of the related literature here serves as a backdrop for the current investigation and helps to understand it in the proper perspective. This can be done in isolation of tasks that have already been done on problems that are directly or indirectly related to the study proposed by a researcher. Do review related literature Prior to any planned research study. The term is also used to describe the written component of a research plan or report that discusses the documents reviewed. In Documents may include articles, abstracts, reviews, monographs, dissertations, books, and other research reports.

Kioumourtzoglou et. al., (1998) aim of this study to assess cognitive, perceptual and motor skill ability in elite Basketball players. Thirteen (n-13) men of elite male national team of Basketball players were selected as a sample for laboratory study aged lies between 22 to 23 years and fifteen men of same age (physical education class) were selected to assess difference in their scores on cognitive skill (memory-retention, memory grouping analytics ability), perceptual skill speed of perception, prediction, selective attention, response selection and motor skills (dynamic balance, whole body coordination, wrist - finger dexterity, rhythmic ability). The result shows that those who are elite Basketball players score better on memory-retention, selective attention, and on prediction measures than the control group.

Ray et. al., (2001) conducted a study to assess the "Effect of yogic exercises on physical and mental health of young fellowship course trainees." The purpose of the study was undertaken to observe the effect of yogic practices during training period on the young trainees. Fifty four trainees were selected for this study. The age lies between 20-25 years. The sample was divided randomly in two groups i.e. yoga and control group. Yoga group (23 males and 5 females) administered yogic practices for the first five months of the course while the control group (21 males and 5 females) did not perform any yogic exercises during this period. From the 6th to 10th month of training both the groups performed the yogic practices. Physiological parameters like heart rate, blood pressure, oral temperature, skin temperature in resting condition, responses to maximal and submaximal exercise, body flexibility were recorded. Psychological parameters like personality, learning, arithmetic and psychomotor ability, mental well being were also recorded. Various parameters were taken before and during the 5th and 10th month of training period. Initially there was relatively higher sympathetic activity in both the groups due to the new work/training environment but gradually it subsided. Later on at the 5th and 10th month, yoga group had relatively lower sympathetic activity than the control group. There was improvement in performance at submaximal level of exercise and in anaerobic threshold in the yoga group. Shoulder, hip, trunk and neck flexibility improved in the yoga group. There was improvement in various psychological parameters like reduction in anxiety and depression and a better mental function after yogic practices.

Bond Dale et. al., (2002) the aim of the study is Moderate aerobic exercise, T'ai Chi,and social problem solving ability in relation to psychological stress. In this study researchers find out the significance of exercise mode, the ability to solve social problems, gender and age in relation to anxiety and difficulties. Samples of the study participants were classified as moderate aerobic exercisers, T'ai Chi exercisers, or seated on the completion of the questionnaire. The ability to solve social problems, the state of anxiety and trait anxiety, and the magnitude and complexity of everyday problems are measured. As predicted, schools demonstrating social problem-solving skills were associated with fewer daily reported problems and lower schools of state concern and factors. For state and trait anxiety, a major effect of exercise mode has emerged after age and sex is under control. A combination of 3 methods including age, gender, and exercise mode suggested that age and gender conveyed the effects of exercise on anxiety, i.e., performance that reduces stress for a variety of exercise modes may depend on a person's age and / or gender. The results of theory, research, and practice are considered.

Dalal (2002) reveals emotion is a motive power, which helps in evolution. In yogic terminology, emotion is a Rajas guna of Prakriti, which exists in everyone. Excitement or upsurge of emotion is responsible for many types of disease. Psycho physiologically, emotions act upon our body through hypothalamus, which controls ANS and the endocrine systems. Negative emotions like anger, fear, greed, jealousy give rise to somatic illness where on the other hand positive emotions like love, compassion, friendship, affection etc. give the strength to combat the stress. Illness due to negative emotions includes hyper acidity, hypertension, insomnia, menstrual disturbances, loss of appetite etc. Daily yoga sadhana of an eight-fold path with a proper balanced diet helps one to act against stressful threshold situations by increasing the threshold of tolerance. The beauty of yoga therapy is that it treats the individual as a whole. An observation was made on 287 sadhakas (male=133 and female=154). Their financial condition, family background and environment were noted. Different symptoms of the subjects were tabulated and studied for every 2 months with the help of physical checkup and psychological testing with different questionnaires related to anxiety, depression, positive and negative outlook towards life. All the findings were again tabulated in detail. The variables stated above were tested before and after the programmes viz., Pratipakshabhavana, Anityabhavana and Sakshibhavana respectively. These practices were done daily for a period of 2 months. The favourable results suggest that Yoga leads to Samadhi, kaivalya, eternal bliss, which aim to maintain physical fitness, mental stability, emotional quietness and spiritual elevation.

Gucray (2003) analysed perceived problem solving skills of secondary students on the basis of some socio-demographic variables. Four hundred ninety eight (n- 498) subjects were selected for this study. In this study Decision Making Scale by Radford et al, 1993 and Problem Solving Inventory by Heppner and Peterson, 1982 used as instruments for data collection. A significant impact of gender, education level, school type was observed on problem solving and decision making of secondary students.

Joshi (2003) study conducted on the effect of some selected yogic practices under the title "Effect of some yogic practice on Human Subject (Physiological and Psychological). The main purpose of the researchers is to find out the effect of Vaman Kriya, Kapalbhati and Bhramari Pranayama on College going students of J.S. Sanskrit Mahavidyalaya, Saptrishi Ashram, Haridwar. Forty male students of 12th standard were chosen as the sample of the study. The age range lies between 18 to 25 years. One hour of yoga training in the morning session was assigned for two months to the students. They performed some yogic practices like Vaman Kriya, Kapalbhati and Bhramari Pranayama. The result of the study shows a significant effect on the students between these Yogic practices. The study shows a significant effect on Haemoglobin, E.S.R., F.V.C, Physical and Mental Health also.

NK, M., & Telles, S. (2004) the purpose of the study was to find out the effect of Spatial and verbal memory test scores following yoga and fine arts camps for school children. The groups of thirty students equally divided into two groups and aged 11 to 16 years were there. One group attended a yoga camp and the other a fine arts camp. Both groups were assessed on the memory tasks pre and after ten days of their respective interventions. A control group (n= 30) was similarly studied to assess the test–retest effect. At the final assessment the yoga group showed a significant increase of 43% in spatial memory scores (Multivariate analysis, Tukey test), while the fine arts and control groups showed no change. The results suggested that yoga practice, including physical postures, yoga breathing, meditation and guided relaxation improved delayed recall of spatial information.

Brown and Gerbarg (2005) evaluate in their studies that the autonomic nervous system, stress related disorders and influencing psychology were balanced by Yogic breathing. In the 1st phase of this study shows the effect of Sudarshan Kriya Yoga (SKY) on neurophysiological theory. Phase 2 shows beneficial and secure usages of yoga breathing on clinical conditions. Results of this study was that SKY was useful post-traumatic stress disorder (PTSD), Stress -related medical illnesses, anxiety, low risk, depression, substance abuse, and rehabilitation of criminal offenders. Mental focus, attention, mood, stress tolerance also improved by yogic techniques. Effect of yoga shows if a professional trainer trained daily for 30 minutes then Patients were motivated by health care providers for yoga practices.

Cowen and Adams (2005) have evaluated the impact of six weeks of either ashtanga Yoga or hatha yoga classes. Significant improvements in follow-up were observed in all participants in diastolic blood pressure, upper body and stem muscle strength and endurance, flexibility, visual stress, and health perception. Progress given by each group compared to basic tests. The group of astanga yoga has lowered diastolic blood pressure and visual acuity, and increased body and stem muscle strength and endurance, flexibility, and a sense of well-being. The development of the hatha yoga group was only important for trunk muscle strength and endurance and flexibility. The findings suggest that the benefits of practicing yoga vary in style.

Fatin (Abdullah) et. al., (2005) investigated physics problem solving skills of secondary students in relation to ethnicity. Five students achieving the highest scores on both the Physics Problems Solving Ability Test (PPSAT) and the Metacognitive Skills Questionnaire (MSQ) were selected to be reassessed using the qualitative techniques. The qualitative techniques are thinking aloud protocol, interviews and analysis of the paper & pencil test by the students. The cross tabulation and triangulation techniques were implied and the results were later being compared with the past researches found in the literature. This study was conducted in Malaysia. It was found that ethnicity has a significant effect on the problem solving ability of secondary students. It was observed that Chinese students have more magnitude of problem solving skills as compared to Malay students but no significant difference was observed in problem solving skills of Indian and Chinese as well as Indian and Malay students. The results showed a partial effect of ethnicity on problem solving skills of secondary students.

Ghaligi, et. al., (2006) revealed in their study that Yogasanas, Meditation and Pranayama helps in raising attention and boosting memory. The group of Chanting showed improvement in scoring of the both memory tests and total error also significantly reduced and the group of non-chanting differed the total time taken for cancellations tests.

Khalsa, et. al., (2006) have evaluated the "Effects of a yoga lifestyle intervention on performance-related characteristics of musicians: a preliminary study". In this study yoga and meditation programs were selected for Musicians enrolled in a prestigious 2-month summer fellowship program at a yoga center. The 10 participants in the yoga program completed baseline and end-program questionnaires evaluating performance-related musculoskeletal conditions, performance anxiety, mood and flow experience. Fellows not participating in the yoga program were recruited to serve as controls and completed the same assessments. Results show that yoga participants showed some improvements relative to control subjects on most measures, with the relative improvement in performance anxiety being the greatest.

Avalle and Vallimurgan (2007) have evaluated the Effects of selected yogic exercise and psychological skill training on selected psycho physiological and psychomotor variables of high- level participants. The sample of the study were selected as forty five intercollegiate level players from Maruthi College of Physical Education, Coimbatore and aged between 18-24 years. The subjects were divided into two variables i.e. psycho-physiological variables and psychomotor variables. The study consisted of a pre – test and post test. The students were divided in three groups: psychological group (PST), yogic exercise (YE) and control group (CG).The psychological group and yogic exercise group practised for twelve weeks and after practiced post tests were conducted. In results, significant differences were found in cognitive anxiety, somatic anxiety, self confidence, heart rate, hand eye co-ordination and reaction time due to influence of yogic exercises and psychological skills training. No significant difference found in case of diastolic blood pressure, systolic blood pressure and body temperature.

Kimbrough et. al., (2007) done a study to assess the "Effect of Inverted Yoga positions on short time memory". In this study, yoga sequence consisting of three inverted positions was designed to test the hypothesis that inverted yoga positions positively influence memory and attention due to increased blood flow to the brain. Three hundred subjects were selected for the study. Solomon four groups design was used for this study. The four groups were designed like; yoga pre/post, yoga post, control pre/post, and control post. All participants completed a short-term memory test of a series of words read aloud at the conclusion of the treatment condition; number of words recalled was the dependent variable. Effect of the testing and treatment was evaluated by ANOVA. In this study, there were no significant differences found between the control group and the experimental group. The practices of inverted yoga position were not affected on short term memory. Any improvement appeared to be the result of being exposed to the pretest rather than the participation in yoga.

Raingruber (2007) The purpose of this study was the effectiveness of Tai Chi, yoga, meditation and Reiki healing sessions in promoting health and enhancing problem solving abilities of registered nurses. Given the current need to retain trained nurses, a self-care program consisting of Yoga, Ti Chi, meditation classes, and Reiki healing sessions is designed for a university hospital. The effectiveness of these interventions was assessed using self-care journals and analyzed using the Heideggerian phenomenological method. The outcomes of the self-care classes described by nurses include: (a) awareness of warmth, tingling, and relaxation, (b) awareness of improved problem-solving ability, and (c) recognition of increased ability to focus on patient needs. Hospitals willing to invest in nursing care options can expect patient and work-related benefits.

Grosse and Simpson (2008) analysed cross-cultural differences in problem solving styles of managers. This study was conducted on two culturally different managers from North American and Latin American origin. Results obtained through Kolb's Learning Style Inventory clearly indicate that Anglo American managers were action oriented and good at decision making as compared to Latin American managers who are more keen on planning and analysing the situation before implementing any decision. It was concluded that managerial problem solving styles differ significantly on the basis of their cultural background.

Dina & Castle (2009) conducted a study on "Analysis of the effect of yoga on selective attention and mental concentration in young adults". This study employed a quasi-experimental pre-test, post-test design to measure whether physical activity had an immediate effect on selective attention and mental concentration in young adults, age of the participants between 18 to 25. This study compared yoga and aerobic exercise classes to assess which one can improve attention yoga practice or aerobic activity. The yoga and aerobic groups completed two surveys and the d2 Test of Attention at two observation points: immediately prior to and immediately following participation in their respective classes. There was significant improvement in pre and post test scores on attention for both groups, as well as greater improvement for the aerobic group.

S.K. Ganguly (2009) recent findings revealed that the study affected the body and mind so Yogic practices are psychophysical. Postural pattern is also known as Aasana. Maharshi Patanjali was described as Asanas in sutras. It indicates that Asanas are psychophysical. Asana is a postural example, which is immovable and agreeable. We can rather say Asanas make dependability and Sukha. We can improve our balance and flexibility with Asanas. Next to the Asanas, Pranayama practices is recommended which requires sitting stable for q uite a while. Since yoga is accepted to be procedure that works with more profound mental thoughtfulness and achieves lasting behavioural transforms, it was viewed as beneficial to survey a portion of these progressions in a logical way.

Subramanya et. al., (2009) aims to determine the Effect of two yoga-based relaxation techniques on memory scores and state anxiety. Fifty seven male volunteers were selected randomly, aged (18-40) were selected for the study. Experimental method (Pre test and post test) designed for the study. Spielberger's State trait Anxiety Inventory (STAI) And Wechsler memory scale (WMS) tools were used for this study. All participants were assessed before and after (i) Cyclic meditation (CM) practiced for 22:30 minutes on one day and (ii) an equal duration of Supine rest (SR) or the corpse posture (shavasana), on another day. Six months of yoga practice involving cycles of yoga postures and supine rest (called cyclic meditation) was previously shown to improve performance in attention tasks more than relaxation in the corpse posture (shavasana). There was significant expandment in the score of all sections of the WMS studied after both cyclic meditation (CA) and shavasana, but the magnitude of alter was more after Cm compared to after savasana. The state anxiety scores decreased after both Cm and shavasana, with greater magnitudes decreased after CM. There was no correlation flanked by percentage alters in memory scores and state anxiety for either section.

Sanjib, B., et. al., (2010) conducted a study examining the effect of yogic actions on psycho-motor variability in physically challenged students. Forty subjects between the ages of 8-15 have been selected for the study. The training program was scheduled for five days a week for 45 minutes each day for six weeks and was increased to 60 minutes weekly in a continuous manner. Further the group was randomly divided into a control and experimental group. Each group had an equal sample size of 20 subjects. Selected psychomotor variants were recorded at the completion and delivery of the 6-week exercise regimen. Psychomotor flexibility data were recorded with the help of standard procedures such as: Speed test motion performed by Nelson and Johnson, Hand stiffness with a fitness test tester and Eye integration with eye-tracking test. This study, therefore, suggests the use of selected yoga practices for students who have been physically challenged. Purpose and objective: The aim and objective of the study was to determine the effect of yogic exercise on selected psychomotor performance namely Speed of Movement, Hand Steadiness and Eye Hand Coordination for physically challenged students. Selected Yogic exercises have been found to be effective in bringing about significant improvements in speed, hand strength and eye coordination for physically challenged students Therefore, research recommends that an additional Yoga Module be developed to improve their psychomotor performance.

Tripathi and Tripathi (2010) this study focuses on the effect of Om (AUM) chanting and Tratak Kriya on concentration ability.The aim of this study to assess the effect of six weeks training program of Om chanting and Tratak on concentration ability. Totally 30 Ph.D Scholars from Banaras Hindu University (BHU) were selected in this study with age range 23-28years .To analyze the collected data paired t-test was applied on said variables and significance level was 0.05 . The results show the significant difference between the before and after means and t- value of concentration ability in the experimental group.In the control group there were no significant differences between before and after the test of mean and t value.

Kumar et. al., (2011) evaluated in their study the effect of yogic pranayama and meditation on selected physical and physiological variables. To accomplish the study purpose 30 boys from Karnataka university department of yoga, Dharwad aged 12-15 years were selected as subjects for this study. The students were divided in two group viz. experimental group and control group. Yogic Pranayama and Meditation were given to the experimental group to do morning and evening alternate days in a week for 12 weeks. No training programme of yoga pranayama and meditation were given to the control group. There were significant improvements shown in the experimental group for the selected physical and physiological factors aside from systolic and diastolic Blood pressure than that of the control group.

Ren J et. al., (2011) conducted the study of meditation promotes insightful problem solving by keeping people in a mindful and alert conscious state. 48 University students with no meditation experience are hired to study the simple meditation process. They were given a list of 10 cognitive problems to solve (the pre-test session). In this study, we focused on unresolved problems and investigated whether they could be successfully solved after 20-minute intervals with or without meditation. Results showed that relative to the control group listening to Chinese or English words, and the language decision-making group, who learned meditation successfully solved more unsuccessful problems from the pre-test session, direct to the role of meditation in promoting insight provided evidence. Further analysis showed that maintaining a mindful and alert state during meditation (raising hands to report every 10 deep breaths compared to every 100 deep breaths), more about failed items from the pre-test session as a result of the information. This implies that it was observable in meditation, rather than relaxation, that actually contributed to the insight. Consistently, in a meditation session or control task, the percentage of alpha waves - the brain index of mental relaxation - was negatively correlated with insight. These results suggest a medita-tion-based insight-promoting mechanism that is involved in passive rest, such as sleep and sleep.

Tasgin (2011) aimed to determine the Problem solving skills of university was explored a study conducted in Turkey. Fifty eight females and eighty six males from Selcuk University, Turkey pursuing a physical education degree were selected as samples. Statistical analysis reveals the female students showed more magnitude of problem solving skills as compared to male students.

Thakur (2011) has evaluated "Immediate effect of Nostril breathing on memory performance". Thirty subjects (boys and girls) were selected for the self control study. Three types of Nostril breathing practices and Breath Awareness effects were tested for this study. Namely verbal recall performance of numerical data such as Digit Span Forward (DSF) and Digit Span Backward (DSB) as well associate learning memory function using Wechsler Memory Scale. Subjects practicing 30 minutes daily, four consecutive days for the interventions included Right Nostril Breathing (RNB), Left Nostril Breathing (LNB), Alternate Nostril Breathing (ANB) and Breathe Awareness. Right nostril yoga breathing (Surya anuloma viloma), there was an increase in digit span toward and digit span backward ($p<0.001$) and alternate nostril breathing also showed significant increase in digit span backward task ($p<0.014$). The LNB effect on the left hemisphere helps to restore the memory function of the right hemisphere. The result shows that the RNB enhances numerical data retrieval mostly as a result of left brain activation.

Amit Kauts (2012) conducted a study on the effect of yoga on concentration and memory in relation to stress. In this study, 800 adolescent students were selected in the beginning; 159 high stress students and 142 low-stress students were selected on the basis of scores obtained through Stress Battery. Two groups are there, one Experimental group and other one control group. Pre test were given to both the groups to assess their concentration as well as short term memory. Experimental group were regularly practicing yoga modules, which consist of asanas, pranayam and prayer for 7 weeks. After the practice post test was also conducted. In this study he revealed that there is improvement in concentration and betterment in short term memory after 7 weeks of yoga modules programme.

Gajjar (2012) have evaluated the effect of Yoga exercises on Academic Achievement, Verbal Reasoning ability and Short-Term Memory (STM) of the students of commerce stream. The single group pre and post design was used for the data collection. The subjects chosen for the study were 40-40 students from two schools. Two groups were divided for the study, one experimental group and second control group. Three tools were used for this study; 1) Academic Achievement test, 2) Verbal Reasoning ability test and 3) Short Term Memory (STM) test. The results show that those who performed yoga are better in academic achievement, improve in short term memory and verbal reasoning ability.

Sharma (2012) the purpose of this study is to assess the effect of yoga modules on Concentration and Memory. For the study, 800 adolescent students were selected, out of which 159 students with high stress, 142 students with from Low stress, on the basis of Stress Battery scores they obtained. The students were divided into experimental group and control group. Pre test was conducted to check students' concentration and short term memory of the experimental group and control group. The experimental group was treated with Yoga modules for seven weeks, whereas no such modules were treated for the control group. Yoga Asana, Pranayama, Meditation, Prayer and Value Oriented Programs are included within the Yoga Module programme. Post test were conducted for both groups (experimental group and control group) to assess their performance on Concentration and Memory tests. The results of the study show that those who performed Yoga modules, improvement in concentration level and boating short term memory.

Bhuyan et. al., (2013) the purpose of this study is to see if yoga has an effect on memory under the stress of an academic exam. The sample consists of 122 Class X students aged 14 to 17, who were randomly assigned to one of two groups. One group did yoga for an hour five days a week, while the control group went about their business as usual. Standard spatial and verbal memory tests were used to assess memory twice during the study: once at the time of enrolment (when no examination stress was present) and again 12 weeks later on the day of the examination

(examination stress). The results demonstrate that the verbal and spatial memory scores are significantly different. The results suggest that yoga improves memory under academic examination stress.

Ebrahimi et. al., (2013) investigated the effect of problem solving strategies on aggression in female athletes. Subjects were divided into two groups: Experimental group and Control group. Experimental groups received a training programme of 12 sessions of Dzurila & Gold fried problem-solving strategies. It was found that after 12 sessions of problem solving training, the experimental group significantly reduced or overcame their aggression in comparison to the control group. It was concluded that other psychological drawbacks are also reduced by problem solving skills.

Gupta (2013) in her study determined the effect of sex and caste on problem solving ability and academic achievement of high school students belonging to scheduled caste and scheduled tribe category. A random sample of 200 students (Boys and Girls) belonging to scheduled tribe and scheduled caste categories was selected from govt. high schools of urban areas of Jammu District. Problem Solving Ability Test prepared and standardized by Dr. L. N. Dubey used this study, while previous years marks were treated as academic achievement. The data was analyzed by (ANOVA). The results revealed that Sex and Caste had significant impact on the problem solving ability of students. No significant difference of sex on the academic achievement of the students and significant impact found of caste on the academic achievement of the students. It was concluded that sex and gender are important markers of problem solving ability of scheduled caste and scheduled tribe high school students.

Yigiter (2013) examined problem solving skills of university students in relation to sports, social activity and demographic variables. Five hundred students from 13 different departments of the university were selected for this study. No sample method was used. Heppner Problem Solving Skill scale was used for the demographic variables and scores of problem solving skills in relation to participants respectively. The findings showed that there was no significant difference between man and female, sport and social activity in preferences, but a significant difference between problem solving skill and demographic variables was found. The demographic variables such as place of residence, father's education, mother's education, age respectively were found to be significantly associated with problem solving skills.

Agashe (2014) a comparative study of hostile aggression between tribal and non tribal sportspersons. This study was conducted on 100 students (50 tribal and 50 non tribal) who participated in inter-university tournaments. Problem solving ability scale prepared by Sharmila and Naga Subramani (2011) was used to collect data. Research found that tribal sportspersons significantly lack problem solving abilities in comparison to non tribal sportspersons. It was concluded that tribal, non tribal culture certainly affects problem solving ability of sportspersons.

Banerjee (2014) aim of the study is to find out the Effect of Yoga on the Memory of Middle School Level Students. Forty (N-40) students of class 7 th from school of Raipur were selected as a sample of the study. Twenty-twenty students were selected in each group (Experimental group and control group). Experimental group practiced yoga regularly in the morning hour's for 60 days. In yoga practices they included Surya namaskar, pranayama, Bhramari, Omkar jap,Yoga nidra etc. P.G.I. the memory scale from N.N.Wing was used to measure memory of the students. The result shows that memory scores between boys and girls also were significantly influenced.

Jena (2014) the purpose of the study is to find out the difference in cognitive styles of undergraduate students in relation to their problem solving ability. This study was conducted on 150 male and 150 female undergraduate students from Pulwama and Anantnag district of J & K. Praveen Kumar's Cognitive Style Inventory and Dubey's Problem Solving Ability Test were used to collect the data. Results reveal significant and positive relationship between cognitive style and problem solving ability. It also demonstrates non significant differences in problem solving ability and cognitive styles of male and female undergraduate students.

Khangholi et. al., (2014) studied the role of problem solving skill training on aggression reduction in athletes. Two hundred twenty (n-220) male basketball players were randomly assigned for this study. There are two groups: Experimental group and Control group. Results shows aggression, hostility including physical and verbal aggression was found to be significantly reduced in male basketball players who took part in problem solving skills training programs.

Khatri and Singh (2014) an experimental study was conducted to see the effect of Kapalbhati and Tratak Kriya on stress and anxiety. The investigator randomly chose a sample of 40 male students aged 18 to 25 years old from the Maharishi Dayanand

University, Rohtak campus for the investigation. The student was enrolled in the university's several teaching departments. The 40 subjects were divided into two groups (group A and group B), each with 20 subjects. Both the group and individual work were given a general warm-up activity. In addition to typical warming up exercises, group was given certain selected yogic kriyas such as shatkarmas, kapalbhati kriya, and tratak kriya. A set of beavers was used as a control group, and they were only given general warming exercises. Both groups received a 9-week training regimen consisting of one hour of training per day in the morning. A stress questionnaire was utilised to determine the subject's degree of stress. The inventory created and standardised by Dr. Rama pal and Dr. Govind Tiwari in 1984 was used to quantify anxiety level anxiety (both state and trait anxiety). The significance of the mean was determined using the T-test. It was discovered that both kriyas, kapalbhati kriya and tractor kriya, have a substantial effect on the psychological components of the students, namely stress and anxiety.

Kolayis et. al., (2014) the aim of this research is to investigate critical thinking and problem solving disposition of athletes. For this investigation 432 athletes (261 male and 171 female) were selected. Problem Solving Inventory and California Scale of Disposition to Think Critically Results show that there was not a significant difference between males and females according to critical thinking. It was found that male athletes had superior problem solving dispositions as compared to female athletes.

Verma (2014) the purpose of this study was to see how yoga practices affected various cognitive development characteristics in adolescent rural residential school students. Eighty-two students, ranging in age from 11 to 15, were randomly assigned to one of two groups: experimental (n= 41) or control (n= 41). In both groups, selected cognitive development characteristics were assessed at the start and completion of a 12-week yoga training programme. In the experimental group, there was a significant improvement in tests of mental capacity and memory. In the control group, however, no statistically significant changes in measures of mental capacity or memory tests were seen. After 12 weeks of yoga training, selected cognitive development characteristics in adolescent rural residential school children improved.

Kumar et. al., (2015) investigates that creative thinking takes the place of problem solving ability which is patterned and framed. It's the ability to think and reason on a given level of complexity. Those who have better problem solving ability are observed to solve the problem of higher 115 complexity faster than those who have more intelligent people. So problem solving ability in young men and women should also be given proper attention by the educationist and trainers.

Ashwathy et. al., (2015) purpose of this study is Effect of Yoga training on Short Term Memory in adolescent age group. Eighty (n-80) school going students aged 11-15 years were selected from Sri Amrutha Vidyalaya, Davangere for this study. There are two groups: Experimental group(40) and Control group(40). Experimental groups performed six months yoga practices for five days a week. Control groups have never performed any training. Pre-test and Post-test" design was utilized. The present study showed that the memory quotient was significantly higher in the yoga trained group compared to the yoga untrained group.

Morteza Taheri (2015) the purpose of this study is to investigate the effect of physical activity on memory and dynamic balance of elder people. The sample of the study were selected as fifteen (n-15) volunteers. The intervention was performed in an eighteen session period, three times a week (each session, 45 minutes). For the mental relaxation they performed Yoga training. Evaluation of memory Wexler test was performed. Dynamic balance was tested by seat ups. The results show that water-based exercises and Yoga protocol have had a positive significant effect on memory ($p=0.03$) and dynamic balance. It was concluded that a selected physical activity program, especially water-based exercises has less potential for making people injured.

Heidari, M., et. al., (2016) aimed to determine the effect of problem solving training on decision- making skill and critical thinking in emergency medical personnel. This study is an experimental study that performed in 95 emergency medical personnel. In this study there are two groups, one control (48) group and experimental (47) group. Experimental group performed a short problem solving course based on eight sessions of 2 hours during the term. Researchers made decision making and California critical thinking skills questionnaires were used for demographic data gathering. The finding revealed that decision -making and critical thinking scores in emergency medical personnel are low and problem solving courses' positively affected the personnel' decision making skill and critical thinking after the education programme.

Shraddha, p., et. al., (2016) revealed a little bit of anxiety is normal; in fact, just like salt in the food, it is needed so that we remain disciplined, focused and aspired. The problem starts when this anxiety becomes so persistent as to start interfering with our daily life, and this is where yoga can help. Sixty (n-60) college going girls (age 17-18 years) was selected as a sample purposely from Nagpur, India. It was found that a significant difference exists between two groups. Results showed that practice of yoga in a day to day life contributes significant enhancement of educational aspiration and considerable reduction of test anxiety.

Mondol (2017) aims to find out Impact of Yoga programs on Reasoning Ability of School going children. Sixty (n-60) students of class 7th were selected as a sample of the study collected from Ausgram High School, Burdwan, and West Bengal, India. The age range of students was between 11to 13 years. The present study was conducted on two groups i.e. Experimental group and Control group. Reasoning Ability was measured before and after 12 weeks of the yoga program in School condition. Reasoning Ability was measured by the Reasoning Ability Test questionnaire developed by L.N. Dubey from National Psychological Corporation, Agra, India and transformed into Bengali versioned by the expert of concerned language. Different variables were calculated by mean and standard deviation and variables were analyzed by applying SPSS. The results show that the impact of Yoga Program on Reasoning Ability was significant.

Joice et. al., (2018) aim of the study is evaluate the influence of yoga in attention, concentration and memory of medical students. The study was conducted on 100 healthy students of medical stream. The age group range was taken between 17-23 years. The twelve week training programme was scheduled and the subjects went through the practice of yoga techniques. The postgraduate institute memory scale was used to measure attention, concentration and memory. The statistically significant improvement was found in attention, concentration and memory of the yoga group. In the control group there was no improvement. This study suggests that after practicing yoga there was a significant improvement in attention, concentration, and memory. These changes may be due to personality development, higher concentration, and reduction of distraction thoughts (mind wandering) due to yoga training.

Jois, S. N., et. al., (2018) in study determined the effectiveness of Superbrain Yoga on concentration, memory and confidence in school students. The concept of

Superbrain Yoga (SBY) is based on ear acupuncture and subtle energy movement in the body. SBY boosts the brain's pranic energy, both qualitatively and quantitatively. The goal of this study is to use SBY to help students enhance their concentration, memory, and confidence. A total of 1,945 pupils from the Mysore district in India participated in the study. For three months, SBY was introduced to kids through their teachers. After three months, the students' responses were gathered using a questionnaire that focused on concentration, memory, and confidence in approaching examinations. The questionnaire's attributes were collected and evaluated using contingency coefficient and Chi-square testing. 86 percent of students said that practising SBY had made them feel more secure when taking exams. Students also said their memory had improved by 75.9% and their focus had increased by 70.5 percent. As a result, SBY has enhanced the school's overall performance.

Shahbazi, S., et. al., (2018) aim of the study was find out the Effects of problem-solving skill training on emotional intelligence of nursing students. A pretest-posttest approach was used in this interventional case–control investigation. The current study included all senior nursing students (n=43) enrolled in the seventh semester of their undergraduate studies at Shiraz University of Medical Sciences' Hazrat Fatemeh School of Nursing and Midwifery. The participants were randomly assigned to one of two groups: intervention (n= 20) or control (n= 23). SPSS software version 16 was used to analyses the gathered data. While the two groups' mean standardized Emotional Quotient Inventory scores were not statistically different before the intervention, the intervention group's scores were significantly higher both immediately and two months later. When standardized emotional intelligence scores were compared to baseline levels, the intervention group had significantly higher mean scores immediately and two months after the intervention (105.879.82 and 109.449.56 vs. 101.2210.93; P 0.001). The control group did not show any significant changes.

Das (2019) have evaluated the Effect of Meditation on Achievement, Attention and Memory of High School students. Two hundred of grade nine high school students (equal no. of boys and girls) were selected for the study. Solomon four group designs were used for subjects. Subjects were divided into four equal groups of 50 students each. Two groups participated in concentration meditation. While in two groups, one participated in meditation, another one did not participate in meditation. Pre test and post test were conducted for all the groups. Odia language ability test, arithmetic test, test for span of attention and test of memory were used to evaluate the achievement, attention and memory. The school examination marks of all participants were collected from school records. After this study it's proven that meditation could be effectively taught to adolescent high school students. The results show significant differences in post-test performance between the meditating and non-meditating groups. The result also established that pre-testing has an impact as the meditating group with pre-testing showed better performance in post-testing among all the groups.

Bhakti et. al., (2020) aimed of the study to Improving Students' Problem Solving Ability through Learning Based Video scribe. The goal of this study is to use media-based video scribe learning to discover problem-solving physics. Students will be more engaging and energetic when they learn with the help of a film because they will be able to understand abstract concepts and solve physics problems that are relevant to their daily lives. The quasiexperimental approach was employed in this study, using a research design of The Randomized Post-Test Only Control Group Design, and 30 students from Indraprasta PGRI University's Physics Education as samples. The T-test was used to analyse the study technique. The findings shown that using learning medium videoscribe to increase problem-solving ability. The findings revealed that using videoscribe as a learning medium can help students enhance their problem-solving abilities in physics. The employment of videoscribe in transmitting physics lectures has considerable favourable effects, according to our findings. Learning is more efficient in physics with the help of video scribe. Pupils are able to understand abstract physics material and engage students in learning. These findings are in line with research on how to increase a student's problem-solving ability in physics class.

Vaezi R (2020) purpose of this study was to investigate the Effect of Yoga on Memory in Elderly Women. Sample of the study were selected by inclusion criteria from to elderly day care centers in Yazd city, in central Iran. In this study control and intervention groups were randomly assigned. Fifty eight (n-58) elderly women were selected and divided in control (n-29) and intervention (n-29) groups. Two months (three 1-h sessions a week) yoga exercises were practiced by an intervention group. The Wechsler Memory Scale was completed for both group's pre and post the intervention. The result shows significant difference in the intervention group but on the other hand there was no significant difference found in the control group. In the intervention group, mental control, logical and visual memory subscales increased significantly (p < 0.05), but there was no significant difference in other subscales. There was no significant difference in any of the subscales in the control group (p > 0.05). Physical activity such as yoga exercise can be helpful for improving the memory of elderly women.

Verma, A., et. al., (2020) aimed to determine the effect of yoga practices on general mental ability in urban residential schoolchildren. Sixty-six urban schoolchildren between the ages of 11 and 15 were chosen as participants. All of the chosen individuals were housed in a residential school in Pune. The students were divided into experimental and control groups using a stratified random sampling procedure. The experimental group had 32 pupils and the control group had 29. At the beginning and end of the 12-week yoga instruction, both the experimental and control groups were examined for general mental capacity using a standard questionnaire. The experimental group received yoga training for 12 weeks, for one hour in the morning, for a total of 12 weeks. During this time, the control group did not get any yoga training. When compared to the control group, the experimental group participants demonstrated a considerable improvement in general mental capacity.

Kallivayalil, J.G., et. al., (2021) the goal of this study was to compare the effects of Yoga and Zumba on memory in the South Indian community in order to raise awareness and better understand the effects of Yoga and Zumba on memory. This was a cross-sectional study of the population of South India. It was distributed to them via a questionnaire. The study's questionnaire had ten items and was distributed to people in South India. The study included a sample size of 100 people, and the data were tabulated appropriately. The information was statistically examined. A total of 100 people took part in the survey. On a daily basis, 75% of the respondents prefer Yoga to Zumba. Yoga, rather than Zumba, can help us control our brains and increase focus, according to 65 percent of respondents. The purpose of this study was to gather information and raise awareness about the effects of Yoga and Zumba on memory in many ways.

Gholam, A. P., et. al., (2021) purpose of the study was to find out the effect of Sudarsankriya yoga practices on P300 amplitude and latency. Adaptive and sustained training can improve cognitive capacity, which was previously thought to be a fixed attribute. Yoga is regarded for sharpening the mind and improving concentration. In order to establish evidences, it is necessary to evaluate the influence of yoga on cognitive ability using objective methods in the early stages of practicing yoga as an alternative/supporting tool to medical treatment. The goal of this study was to record and compare peak latency and amplitude to see how regular practise of sudarsankriya yoga affected auditory event related potential (P300). Group I and Group II were the first and second groups, respectively. The participants were divided into three groups, with Group I practising sudarsankriya yoga for more than 36 months and Group II practising sudarsankriya yoga for less than 36 months, respectively. Non-practitioners in Group III have never done any sort of yoga before. The study enlisted 20 volunteers in each group, for a total of 60 participants ranging in age from 40 to 65. Between the three groups, there was a significant variation in mean latency and amplitude. The current study's findings imply that sudarsankriya yoga practise delays the ageing process or maintains cognitive abilities in adults.

Swaroop, S. et. al., (2021) have evaluated the Effect of Yoga Exercise on Achievement, Memory and Reasoning Ability. One hundred students of class 11th (U.P. Board and C.B.S.E. Board) were selected as a sample of the study. Field Experimental Method was used for the study. Academic Achievement Test and Short Term Memory test was used as a tool of the study. The result shows that yoga exercise improves the memory and academic achievement of the students.

CHAPTER 3

METHOD AND PROCEDURE

This chapter describes selection of subjects, selection of variables, criterion measure, reliability of data, experimental design, collection of data, procedure for administration of tests, and statistical techniques.

The research methods and procedure followed in this study are mentioned in this chapter. To conduct research from the initial identification of the problem to the conclusion, the researcher employs specific methods and follows all procedures in a systematic manner. The research methods provide the tools and techniques with which the problem will be addressed.

It includes the methods and procedures that will be used in the study in a certain order. This chapter explains the selection of subjects, selection of variables, criterion measure, reliability of data, experimental design, collection of data, procedure for administration of tests, and statistical techniques used to investigate the Effect of Yoga on Memory and Problem-Solving Ability of Players.

3.1 RESEARCH METHODS

3.1.1 Design

The study is an experiment one, where pre and post test designs have been followed. Four groups of the students were selected and given specific yogic exercise with general warm up. All four groups were given some selected yogic asana. All the four groups have been pre-tested and post tested, for selected psychological components (Memory and Problem-Solving Ability). The change in the variable or say components is credited to the exercise to the groups.

3.1.2 Sample and Training Programme

In the present study purposive sampling procedure has been followed. A group of hundred (boys and girls) students studying in graduation and post graduation have been selected from the different universities of Haryana i.e. Chaudhary Devi Lal University (CDLU), Sirsa; Chaudhary Ranbir Singh University (CRSU), Jind; Kurukshetra University, Kurukshetra (KUK); Maharshi Dayanand University (MDU),

Rohtak. The age group range lies between 20 to 25 years. Furthermore, these one hundred four students have been divided equally into 4 groups on the University basis, consisting of 25 students each. Here all groups have gone through common yoga protocol exercise for two hours daily during morning and evening sessions for 6 days per week during four weeks training programme under strict supervision of the researcher.

3.1.3 Selection of Subjects

The study was carried out on 100 (50 boys and 50 girls of group 20 to 25 year) at university level, players from four universities of Haryana and the data was collected randomly from yoga camp of different participants of Inter University yoga camp. The pre and post group design of yoga players were used for this study.

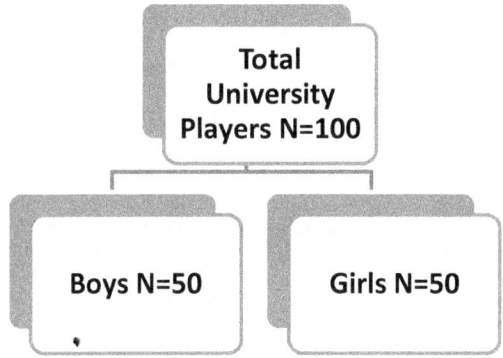

Figure 1: Flow chart of study Design

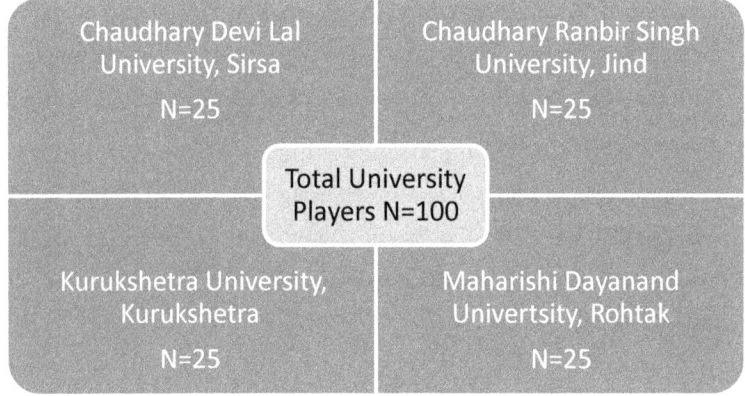

3.1.4 Selection of Variables

The Research Scholar gleaned through all the scientific literature pertaining to Yoga from books, magazines, journals, periodicals. The Research Scholar discussed with experts of this field, keeping in view the feasibility of criterion and the relevance of study for the following variables which were selected. To compare the four groups (Chaudhary Devi Lal University, Sirsa; Chaudhary Ranbir Singh University, Jind; Kurukshetra University, Kurukshetra; Maharishi Dayanand University, Rohtak) various components from psychological area: Memory (remote memory, recent memory, mental balance, attention - concentration, delayed recall, immediate recall, retention for dissimilar parts, visual retention and recognition) and Problem Solving Ability Test were selected. The components were selected by keeping in view their significance from a performance point of view.

Main variables chosen are as following:

- Independent Variable

    Yoga

- Dependent Variable

    Memory

    Problem Solving Ability

3.1.5 Criterion Measures

- Memory was assessed by a memory scale PGI Memory Scale (PGIMS) constructed by D. Pershad and N.N. Wig (1977). It contained 10 sub-test- remote memory, recent memory, mental balance, attention - concentration, delayed recall, immediate recall, retention for dissimilar parts, visual retention and recognition.

- Problem Solving Ability was assessed using students' examination problem solving ability tests by L.N. Dubey (1971). This test was consisted of 20 problems. Each problem had four alternative answers. The duration of this test was 40 minutes.

3.1.6 Experimental Design

The pre and post-test randomized groups design was adopted for this study. All the subjects were divided into four groups each comprising 25 subjects. Each group had students of equal status with respect to age, diet, socio economic conditions. Further, the experimental treatments were also assigned randomly to all experimental groups. All the groups were assigned specific yogic training programmes consisting of Asanas, Pranayamas and Suryanamaskar and Kriya after general warming up. The training was carried out for a total duration of four weeks. The subject voluntarily participated in the study. All the four groups were pre-tested as well as post tested on the selected components of psychological areas.

3.2 RELIABILITY OF DATA

The reliability of data was assured by establishing the instrument reliability, tester competency and reliability of tests and subject reliability.

Instrument Reliability

PGI Memory Scale constructed by D. Pershad and N.N Wig (1977) and Problem Solving Ability Test developed by L.N. Dubey (1971) were used in this study.

Test -retest was used to find out the reliability for PGIMS by N.N. Wig was .70 and .84 for the organic-psychotic group and between .48 and .84 for the neurotic-normal group. For PSAT the test-retest reliability range between .7.

Reliability of the PGI memory scale test by D. Pershad and N.N. Wig (1977)

Paired Samples Correlations				
		N	Correlation	p-value
Pair 1	PGI Test & PGI Re-Test	25	0.791	0.001**

The above table explains the reliability of the test and the coefficient of the reliability was calculated using Spearman-Brown formula. As per the figures of the above table, the correlation coefficient is 0.791, and the p-value is 0.001, which indicates that the correlation coefficient was highly significant. Since, the coefficient value was greater than 0.7; hence, the PGI memory scale test was highly reliable.

Reliability of the Problem-Solving Ability Test (L.N. Dubey 1971)

Paired Samples Statistics

Paired Samples Statistics							
		N	Mean	Std. Deviation	Std. Error Mean	t-value	p-value
PSAT	PSAT Test	25	10.400	2.739	0.548	1.825	0.080
	PSAT Re-Test	25	11.040	2.835	0.567		

The above table exhibits the output of the paired t-test which was applied to investigate the difference in the results of problem-solving ability test (PSAT), before and after attending the yoga camp. The purpose of the test was to determine whether there was statistical evidence and the mean difference between paired observations was significantly different from zero. As per the above table, t-value 1.825 and p-value 0.080 (p-value>0.05) indicates that the p-value was not strong enough to reject the null hypothesis, hence we accept the null hypothesis that there was a non-significant difference in the results of the problem-solving ability test (PSAT) and re-test. Figure 1 shows the mean of the problem-solving ability test (PSAT) for all respondents, before and after attending the yoga camp.

Reliability of the problem-solving ability test (PSAT) (L.N. DUBEY 1971)

Paired Samples Correlations				
		N	Correlation	p-value
PSAT	PSAT Test & PSAT Re-Test	25	0.803	0.001**

The above table explains the reliability of the test and the coefficient of the reliability was calculated using Spearman-Brown formula. As per the figures of the above table, the correlation coefficient was 0.803, and the p-value was 0.001, which indicates that the correlation coefficient was highly significant. Since, the coefficient value was greater than 0.7; hence, the problem-solving ability test (PSAT) was highly reliable.

The reliability scores of the tests used in the study were accepted as accurate enough for this study.

3.2.1 Validity

The coefficient of validity was calculated by correlating the scores with the Problem Solving Ability Test developed by the L.N. Dubey (1971) 0.68 to 0.85.

3.3 PROCEDURE FOR DATA COLLECTION

Data "collection was essentially an important part of the research process so that inferences, hypotheses or generalizations tentatively held may be identified as valid, verified as correct or rejected as untenable." Collection of information of data requires a systematic procedure, because as per Whitney (1964), "Data are the things we think with. They were the raw materials of reflection until by comparison, combination and evaluation they were stepped up to higher levels of generalization, where again they serve as basic material for further and higher thinking." It also requires collection of relevant data adequate in quality and quantity and as reliable and valid as possible.

In the beginning, all 100 players studying in the different universities of Haryana selected for the present study was administered both tests as per standardized instructions given in the manual. The tools were administered at each subject of all groups individually for pre-test and post-test. They were tested when they were performing yoga exercises. The Problem Solving Ability test was distributed to the same 100 players of different universities. The investigator explained to all the participants, the instructions and way of answering the question. The time limit for the test was only 40 minutes. This was a well standardized test with established norms which were tabulated in the manual with full procedural details. The students were asked to fill the columns of personal particulars before the test started.

The PGI Memory Scale contains 10 sub-test- remote memory, recent memory, mental balance, attention - concentration, delayed recall, immediate recall, retention for dissimilar parts, visual retention and recognition. Test were constructed with simple sentences and questions that could be easily administered.

The students were asked to fill the columns of personal particulars before the test started.

It had one separate answer sheet as students had to mark their responses given on the sheet. There were 15-20 minutes time limit for answering the PGI Memory Scale, but they were asked to complete it as early as possible. While administering the test, the investigator paid sincere attention via supervision.

After the administration of 'Problem solving ability (PSAT)' by L.N. Dubey (1971), PGI Memory Scale (PGIMS) constructed by D. Pershad and N.N. Wig (1977) were administered. The test material goes into four parts: (a) Test Booklet (reusable) (b) Answer sheet for answering (c) Scoring key for evaluating the answer and (d) Test Manual for direction and table of conversion.

In the beginning, when all the students were seated, the procedures for answering the multiple-choice items were explained verbally. Then the test paper was distributed among the testes and they were instructed to fill in their name and other items required for the title page of each test. For this, only five minutes were given for each test. Then the testes were asked to read the instructions on the title page of the test very carefully. When each testes was done with all this, the administrator asked if there were any doubts regarding the test. They were also told the maximum time limit for completing the test.

The investigator clarified all the doubts and then the testes started the test. When the time limit was over, the test papers were collected. Before receiving the sheets the administrator made sure that the necessary information had been done in the blanks of the achievement test. The investigator assured the students that their answers and scores would be kept in confidence. While administering all tests, the time limit was strictly followed as per the instruction. The investigator was sincere attentive at the time of administering the test. To summarize, the whole procedure for data collection; in the initially 100 players selected from different universities were administered for the test for PGI Memory Scale and Problem Solving Ability Test (PSAT). Scoring of each test was done strictly according to the norms of the respective test.

3.3.1 Procedure for Administration of the Test

PGI Memory Scale by D. Pershad and N.N. Wig (1977)

Objective

To measure the memory of the participants.

Equipment

Paper Pencil

Description

Subjects were well explained before filling up the questionnaire and each subject was given a pen along with the questionnaire. In case of any doubt regarding the statement the researcher clarified the same to the subjects. Filling up the questionnaire took only 15-20 minutes and it was collected back after being filled up.

Scoring

PGI Memory Scale contains 10 sub-tests- remote memory, recent memory, mental balance, attention-concentration, delayed recall, immediate recall, retention for dissimilar parts, visual retention and recognition. After scoring of each sub tests, the scores were added for total score of the full test. The maximum possible score for the full test was 115.

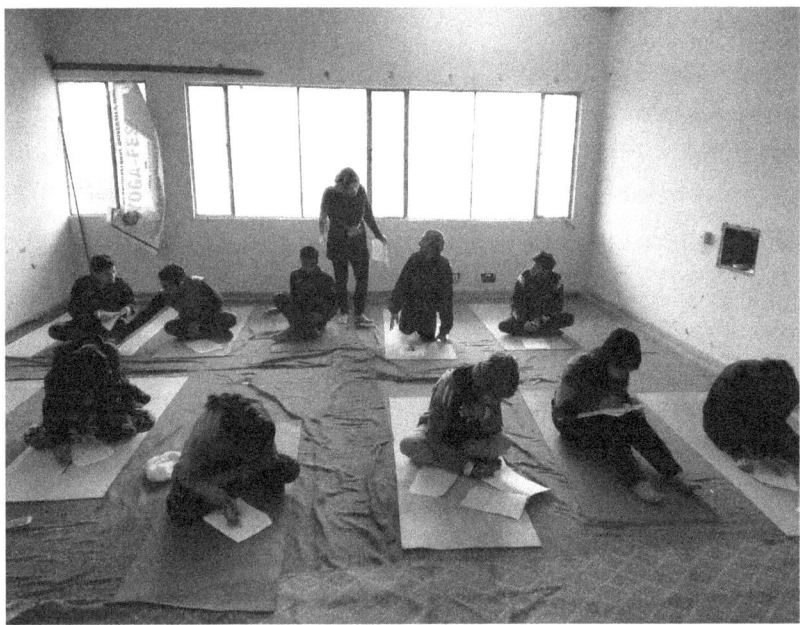

3.3.2 Problem Solving Ability Test by L.N. DUBEY (1971)

Objective

To measure the Problem-Solving Ability of the participants

Equipment

Paper Pencil

Description

To measure the Problem-Solving ability of the subjects, the first test was conducted before the beginning training program. It was administered again after completion of the training program. For the conduct of the test, players were distributed a problem-solving ability test. They were asked to mark the correct answer in the test. The total time for the test was 40 minutes. It was instructed to the player that maximum attempts should be made within stipulated 40 minutes time.

Scoring

Each problem had four alternative answers. Out of four answers one was correct. If the player writes the correct answer he/she should be given one mark, if the answer was wrong then they get zero marks. The duration of this test was 40 minutes.

To measure

This test enabled us to measure the problem-solving ability in order to plan our training programme to develop it by providing adequate training and practice. This test also had productive value. Problem-solving abilities were highly correlated with intelligence, reasoning ability and mathematical ability.

3.4 ADMINISTRATION OF TRAINING PROGRAMME

The training for the experimental group was administered at Yoga hall of different universities of Haryana. The experimental group came for six days in a week for the period of four weeks and each experimental session was for two hour duration. Subjects were briefed about the training programme. All the groups of students participated in the training programme.

3.4.1 Contents of the training programme for each experimental group were given below:

Only those training programmes were used for the study which were recommended by Association of Indian Universities for the Inter-University of Yoga Championship.

Description of Asanas Practice

The first step was to attain the asana posture. In this phase the movements should be synchronized, balanced, step by step and self controlled.

The second step was to retain the posture for prescribed duration. While doing yogic posture you should be comfortable, safe and calm with no shivering movements.

The third step was to return from the posture which we gain during asana practices. In this step also, our movement should be synchronized, rhythmic, step by step and controlled.

Throughout the practice, the emphasis should be on achieving stability for a set period of time in each asana; the next stage was to feel comfortable in this position. It was important to be able to hold the asana comfortably and with ease.

General Instructions and Precautions:

I) Person who has a history of any chronic and serious illness should tell the yoga teacher before starting yoga practice.

II) People suffering from back pain, neck pain, spondylitis, high blood pressure, heart disease, slip disc, diabetes, cancer etc. should practice yoga under the supervision of an expert yoga teacher. However, in the present study the subject has not been found to suffer from such problems.

III) Asanas should be done on an empty stomach and there should be a gap of 5 hours between meals and exercises.

IV) All phases of asana I. e. Attaining the posture, maintaining the posture and returning from the pose should be performed in a synchronized and rhythmic motion.

V) Avoid jerky movements, otherwise it may cause injury.

VI) Initially during asana practice, practitioners may feel body pain and muscle stiffness. Do not worry and practice asana regularly, the pain will disappear gradually.

VII) For a novice practitioner, it was not possible to achieve the correct posture, so in this case the practitioner should remain in the posture obtained after a lot of effort.

VIII) In the early stages, a novice practitioner will face difficulty breathing in most of the asanas after attaining the final posture, so the practitioner should take short breaths during posture retention.

IX) If the practitioner feels very uncomfortable while maintaining the posture, the practitioner should slowly release the posture without jerking, rest for some time (a few seconds) and start again.

X) In the beginning, the practitioner may suffer from muscle cramp due to abnormal muscle contractions. In such a situation, after returning from the posture, massage the muscle, rest for some time and start the practice again.

3.4.2 Selected Asanas During The Training Program is Given Below

Ardha Badh Padmottanasana

Bakasana (Urdhva Kukkutasana)

Chakrasana

Dhanurasana

Ekapad Rajkapaotasana

Ekapada Shirshasana

Halasana

Hanumanasana

Karna Pidasana

Mayurasana

Natarajasana

Paschimottanasana

Purna Bhaujangasana

Purna Chakrasana

Purna Dhanurasana

Purna Matasendrasana

Purna Shalabasana

Sarvangasana

Setubandh Sarvangasana

Sirsasana

Titiabhasana

Ustrasana

Vajrasana

Vatayanasana

Vrischikasana

Kriya (Jal Neti, Sutra Neti)

Pranayama

Nadishodhan Pranayam

Bhramari Pranayama

Kapalbhati Pranayama

Surya Namaskar

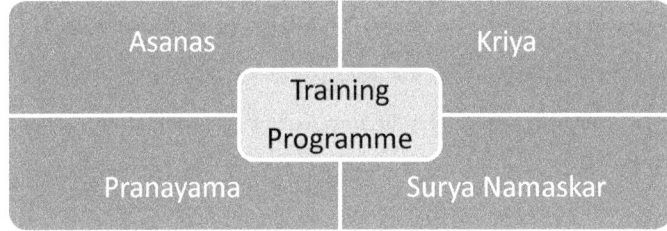

ARDHA BANDH PADMOTTANASANA

- First, stand in tadasana or mountain pose.
- Inhaling lift your left leg and bring the left foot on the right thigh and bring it as much as possible.
- In this posture, you will stretch on your left hip and knee.
- If the foot is sliding downward, then you can hold it with the right hand.
- Now take your left hand from the back and hold the left toe.
- lean the joints of the hip, leaving the breath be careful not to the waist or knee joint.
- Breath while bending down.
- Place your left hand on the ground beside your left foot.
- Take five breaths in total and leave them out, so that you can stay in the asana for 30 to 60 seconds.
- Try to keep your back straight and keep the left leg straight.
- Let your hand hang tight so that your neck muscles are not stressed.
- After practices, the asana on the left side, repeat all the steps on the other side too.

BAKASANA (URDHVA KUKKUTASANA)

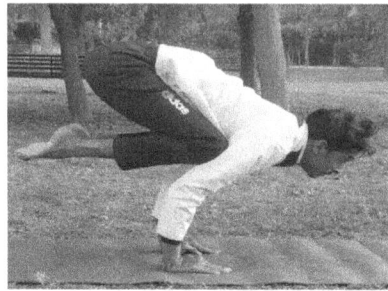

- Bend your knees and place your hand to the floor, shoulders width apart.
- Lean forward a little to bring the knees close to the armpits as much as you can.
- Transfer your body weight to your arms, completely while your toes are still on the floor.
- Gently Press your knees against the arms and slowly lift your big toes off the floor.
- Raise your buttocks a little and balance the body slowly on your arms.
- Lift your head, lengthen your neck.
- Lift straight to focus your gaze on a fixed point.
- Once you have secured the balance, put your feet together.
- Breathe normally and hold the position for 5 to 15 breaths.
- To come out of the pose slowly lower your feet to the floor.
- Relax the body by taking low and deep breaths.

DHANURASANA

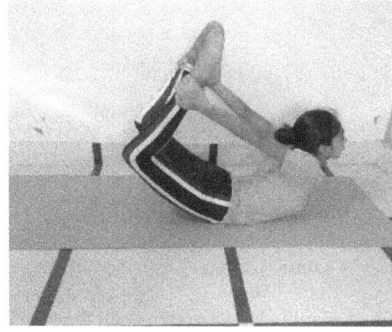

- Lie flat in a prone position with the legs and feet together.
- Take a deep breath and exhale, bend your knee such that your heels touch the hips and hold the ankles with your hands.
- Move slowly and with control as you inhale.
- Arch the back lifting the thigh,head,thorax and hip together.
- Try to balance the body weight on the lower abdomen.
- Stretch your neck backward and look forward; try to join the ankles and start normal breathing.
- Hold the pose for one minute.
- Now the exhalation comes down. Now release the hand grip from the ankle and slowly lower the leg, chest and head.
- At last you should relax for one minute.
- Practice up to 2 rounds.

EKAPADA SHIRSHASANA

- With your legs straight, sit comfortably in the Staff Pose (Dandasana).
- After that, twist (bend) your right knee slightly. Now, with your left knee, keep the sole of your right foot on the floor.
- Lower your right knee to the right side of the floor as the next step. Open your hips now.
- The crucial factor for setting up the final position is hip movement or rotation.
- After then, grab/hold your right foot's ankle. Take your right shin and hug it to your chest.
- However, you must keep your ankle parallel to the other.
- Simply hold your right ankle with your left hand and pull it towards you.
- Now comes the difficult part: carefully lift and bring your right knee towards your shoulder.
- You must place your right ankle behind the neck and your left shoulder.
- If your leg contacts your neck, you can lean forward for a few seconds to keep the position.

- Maintain the straightness of your other leg in front of you. It's worth noting that your sit bones are firmly planted.
- On the top of your shoulder, move your right shoulder forward and your right leg backward.
- When your right foot feels entirely tucked behind your neck.
- Then make a prayer stance by bringing both hands to your chest (Namaste gesture). Your hands, however, should be touching your chest.
- Now that you've reached the final position, hold it for five to six breaths.
- Lower your hands and grip the right toe with your left hand.
- Your right leg should be unfolded and lowered.
- Carry on in the same manner with your other leg.

EKAPAD RAJAKAPOTASANA

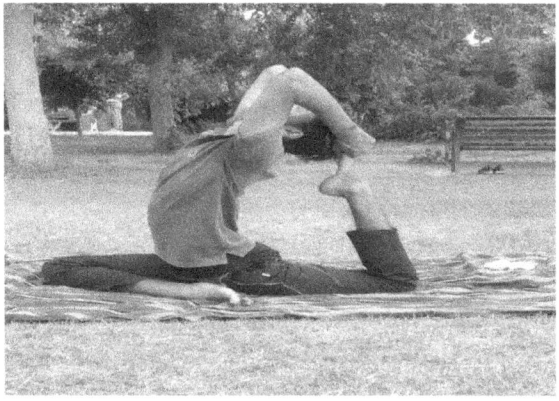

- Bend your left knee and place your left foot towards your right waist, toes touching. Straighten your right leg, keeping the front of your thigh, shin, and top of your foot on the floor. Square your hips to the front and widen your right hip to the right.
- Backwards extend your right hand, palm facing up. Inhale and stretch your arms and legs out to the sides of your body. Exhale and turn to the right with your head, torso, chest, and shoulders. Bend your back leg and reach out with your right hand

to grab your right leg. Turn your leg out to the side and take a firm grip on the instep.

- keep your torso and shoulder to the right. Exhale and bring the right side of your torso and shoulder forward, keeping your elbows straight. Take a deep breath and bend your right elbow upward. Rotate the arm and bring the palm down while keeping a strong grip on the foot. Distribute the weight evenly between the left hip and the front of the right thigh by pressing the fingers of your left hand down. Build a firm, balanced base by drawing from your knees into the centre of your pelvis.

- Inhale and rise from your waist to your shoulders, pressing your left fingertips to the floor. Bring your upper arms parallel and your elbows closer together. Pull your elbows back toward your shoulders, hollowing out your armpits as you do so. Reach your left arm up and back and grip your leg while exhaling. To intensify the shoulder stretch, press your right foot against the resistance of your hands. Lift your chest behind your heart and draw your shoulder blades into your back.

- Tilt your head back until your right foot is in contact with it. Stay in the stance for a few breaths before exhaling and lowering your leg one by one. Repeat on the opposite side.

HALASANA

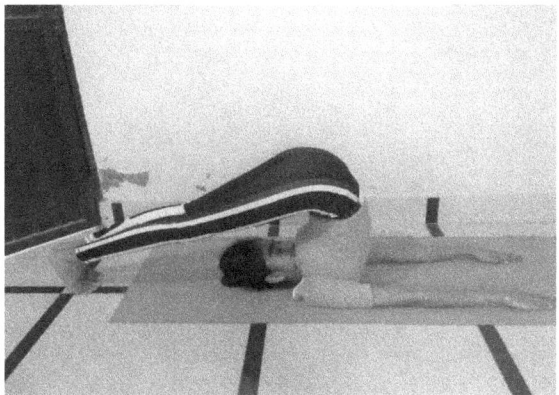

- Lie down on the floor in supine position, with stretched arms close to the body in pronation position, keep the palms flat on the ground.

- Join the legs together and stretch the knees straight.

- Inhale as in complete deep breathing and exhale slowly; raise the leg slowly vertically to an angle of 90 degree.
- Press the arms and palm on the ground and raise the waist and both the legs upwards; then bend the legs forward towards heads by curving the back then try to touch the ground behind head.
- Breathe slowly and stretch the legs away from the head and legs should be straight.
- The whole weight will lie on the shoulder and try to stretch the supine straight in an upward direction.
- Hold the posture for one minute.
- Now slowly release pose to return to initial position.
- Relax completely for one minute with deep breathing.
- Repeat the process twice.

HANUMANASANA

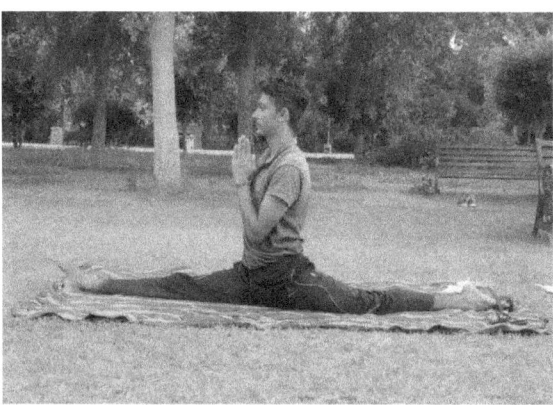

- To begin, kneel on your left knee.
- Place your right foot next to your left knee.
- Without exerting undue pressure, slowly slip the left foot backward and the right foot forward. Legs should be moved as far backwards and forwards as possible.
- Now, use your hands to balance the weight of your body.
- Attempt to place your buttocks on the floor.

- Relax your entire body.
- Put your hands in front of your chest and clasp them together.
- Hold this position for one minute.
- Slow down your breathing. Slowly and comfortably inhale and exhale.
- The same asana repeats with the right leg pointing backward.

KARNAPIDASANA

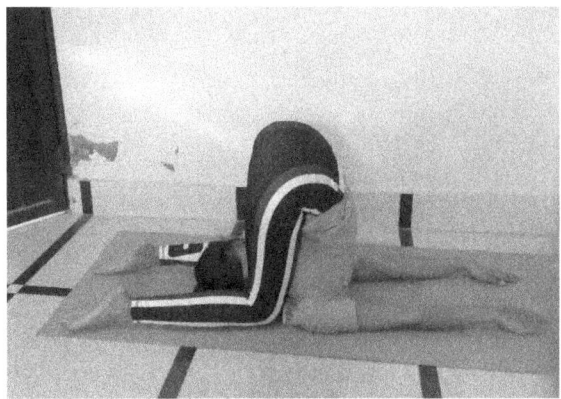

- Lay down in a spine position on the floor.
- Keep both hands and feet in a straight line.
- Then take a deep breath and raise the legs slowly toward the sky.
- After this try to move your legs slowly behind the head.
- Keep the entire weight of your body on the shoulders. During this time your hand should be straight on the ground as before.
- This is the situation of halasana, now bend both your legs on your knees.
- After turning both knees, they will come near the ears. This will cover both the ears from the knees. In this situation, you keep your eyes on the nose.
- Stay in this same posture for one minute and keep breathing at normal speed.
- Then slowly reverse this Aasana while exhaling to get to the starting position.
- Practice two more times for this asana.

MAYURASANA

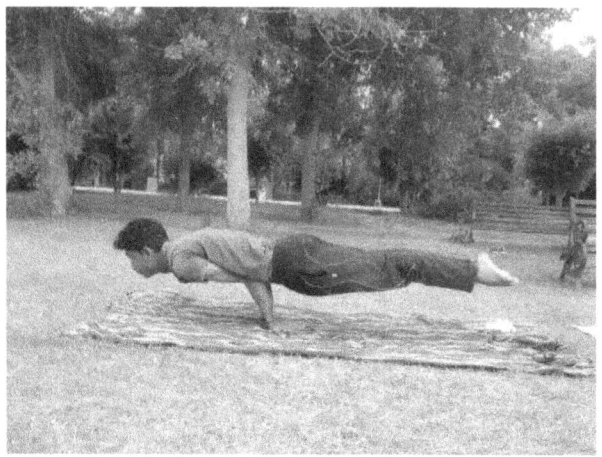

- Sit with your knees bent on a flat surface.
- Make sure your knees are wide apart and your heels are near to one other.
- Knee forward and place your palms on the ground between your knees, directing your fingers toward your torso.
- Bend your elbows gently and press them towards your abdomen, placing your entire body weight on your hands.
- Stretch your legs rearward slowly, lifting them off the ground.
- Your entire body should be above and parallel to the ground in the ultimate posture, with all of your body weight on your hands and arms.
- Set your eyes forward by tightening your shoulders, straightening your head, and tightening your shoulders.
- Hold the pose for a few minutes, but don't force it. Gently return to your original position.
- Relax your body and take calm, deep breaths in and out.
- At least three times, try to repeat this asana. You may, however, practice it according to your abilities.

NATARAJASANA

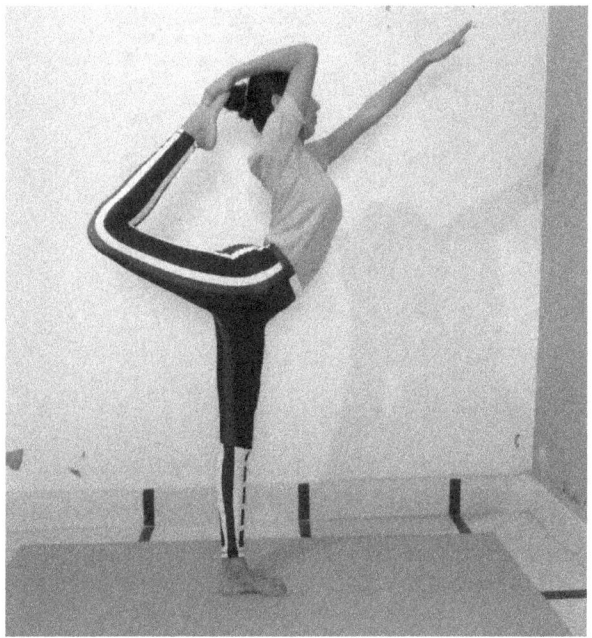

- Relax the body in mountain pose and breathe normally.
- Bend the right knee to raise the leg toward the buttock. Hold the right big toe with the right hand.
- Maintain your body weight on the left leg. Next raise your right leg backward as far as you can.
- While your body weight on your left leg, relax your shoulders so that the elbow of the right arm points upwards.
- Now raise your left leg arms upward. Keeping the hand straight with the palm facing downward.
- Balance your body along while maintaining your gaze if comfortable, breathe normally.
- Hold the pose from 20 second to 1 minute, gradually increasing the time each day.
- Practice 2 to 3 times, evenly on each side by changing the position of leg and arms.

PURNA DHANURASANA

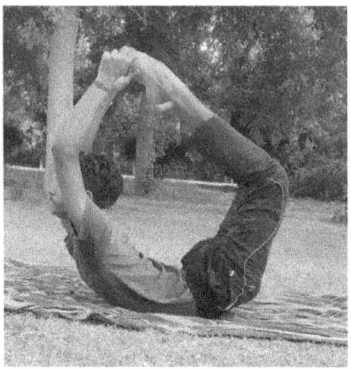

- Lie straight on the stomach.
- Bend both the knees. Clasp both the feet with the hands.
- Inhale deeply and raise the head, chest and thighs as high as possible. Furthermore, pull the feet as close to the head as possible. Keep the elbows pointing upward.
- Now, the body seems to resemble a fully stretched bow. Retain the breath inside and hold in the same position for as long as comfortable.
- Return to the earth by slowly exhaling and releasing both legs.
- Relax your entire body until your breathing and heartbeat are regular again. The first round has concluded.
- It is usually adequate to practice just one round of this asana. When done before or after any forward bending asana, it is more effective.

PASCHIMOTTANASANA

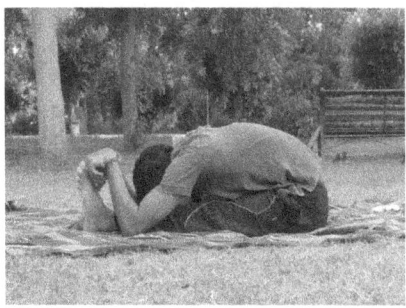

- Begin with sitting with legs stretched out in front of you with a deep inhale.
- Keep the spine erect and toes flexed toward you.
- Raise both hand arms above your head and stretch up, straight beside the ears.
- Now exhale the breath and keep the spine erect, focusing on moving forwards towards the toes.
- Hold the toes of your legs with the index and middle fingers of both the hands.
- With a normal breathing process, bend as much forward as one can and should try to touch the floor with elbows besides the knee joints. Now your face is in between the legs on shin bones for some time.
- Maintain this pose for some time.
- Come back to the initial position and lower the arms and relax completely for 1 minute with deep breathing.
- Practice up to 2 rounds is enough.

PURNA MATASENDRASANA

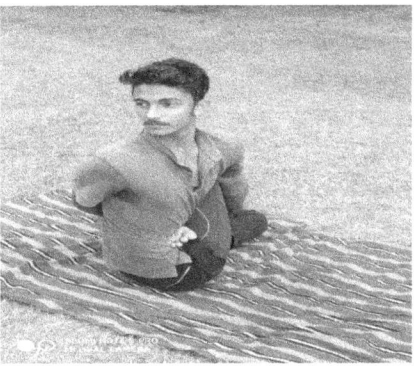

- Firstly, lie down in a prone position. Your forehead should be relaxed and resting on the ground.
- Keep your legs joined together and keep your arms near the body.
- Keep your hands beside the chest, palms pointing to the ground.
- Now inhale and slowly raise your upper body along with your chest, till the navel.
- Now exhale and bend your spine backward.

- Release your neck.
- Hold this position for at least thirty seconds.
- Now gradually raise your legs while bending your knees and attempt to get your feet as close to your head as possible.
- For thirty seconds, try to stay in this position.
- Exhale and return to your original position.
- Now take a rest for sixty seconds.
- Repeat this process for 2-3 times in one session.

PURNA CHAKRASANA

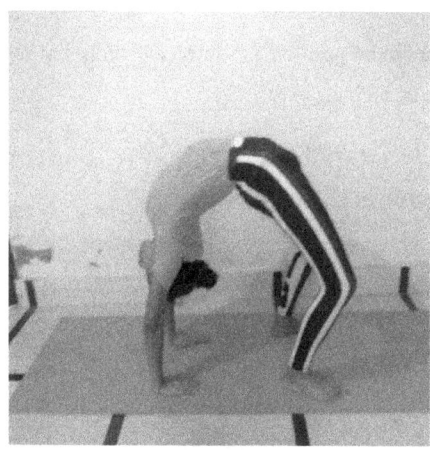

- Lie down in Supine position on the ground.
- Bend your knees and bring your heels closer to touch your hips. Keep some distance between your feet.
- Now raise your hand and bring your palms under your shoulders in such a manner that the fingers point towards the shoulder and elbow point towards the sky.
- Now while inhaling, press your palms of both hands and feet on the ground and lift your body upward direction.
- Now try to lift your body upward to the maximum possible level through the induction of optimum stretching and tension in the body.

- In this position, the spine rolled like a semi-circular figure. Thorax, abdomen and pelvis are pushed upward and head point towards the ground.
- Perform Chakrasana first.
- Slowly exhale, then move your palms towards your heels.
- Keep the crown of the head close to your hips.
- Hands and legs should be solid and stretched out perfectly.
- Continue to hold this position for 8 to 10 seconds, breathing evenly.
- Now release your pose slowly to come to the starting position.
- Relax for a few moments and then repeat almost 2 to 4 times more throughout a yoga session.

PURNA BHUJANGASANA

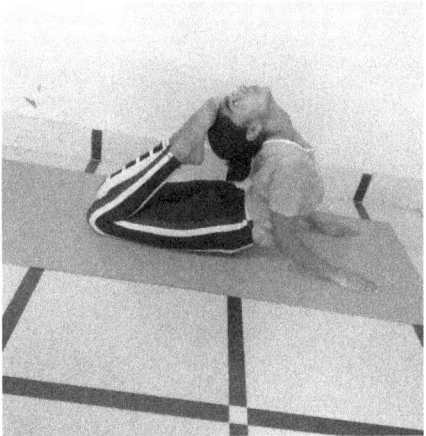

- Lie down on your stomach first. Your forehead should be relaxed and laying flat on the earth.
- Keep your legs together and your arms close to your torso.
- Keep your palms pointing to the ground and your hands beside your chest.
- Inhale now and slowly elevate your upper body, including your chest, to your navel. (A soft and leisurely movement is preferable to a jerky movement.)
- Now take a deep breath and bend your spine backward.

- Now release your neck.
- Hold this position for at least thirty seconds.
- Now gradually raise your legs while bending your knees and attempt to get your feet as close to your head as possible.
- Try to touch your head with your toes. (as much as possible)
- Hold this position for at least thirty seconds.
- Breathe out (exhale) and return to your starting posture (slowly down your legs first, and also the torso).
- Now take a sixty-second break.
- In one session, repeat this method 4 to 5 times.

SARVANGASANA

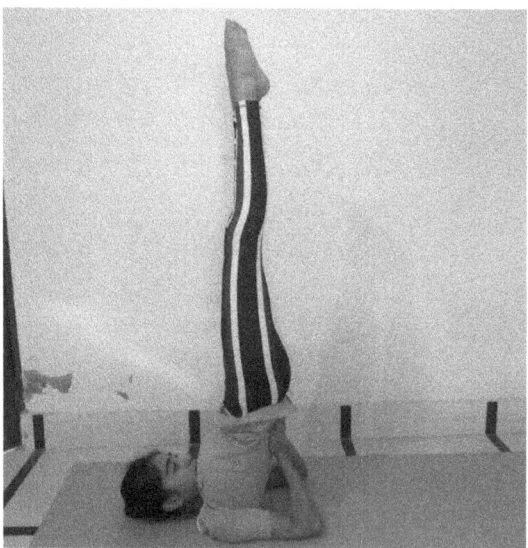

- Lie down on the floor in supine position. Hands should be below the hip, arm facing upward, elbow close to the body, you may tuck the elbows below the back. As you exhale, bend the knees and lift the hip off the floor.
- Inhale, straight in the legs, turning them straight.
- Placing the elbows closer to each other will help Protect the back and give more stability. Hold this position as much as you can.

- Exhale bend the knees toward the chest.
- Inhale with the help of the hands and bring the hip down.
- You may unbend the knees as you come down to help maintain the center of gravity to control the motion. When you come down make sure you don't come down with a jerk. It's very important to come down slowly. Relax completely with deep breathing for one minute.
- Repeat the process twice.

SIRSASANA

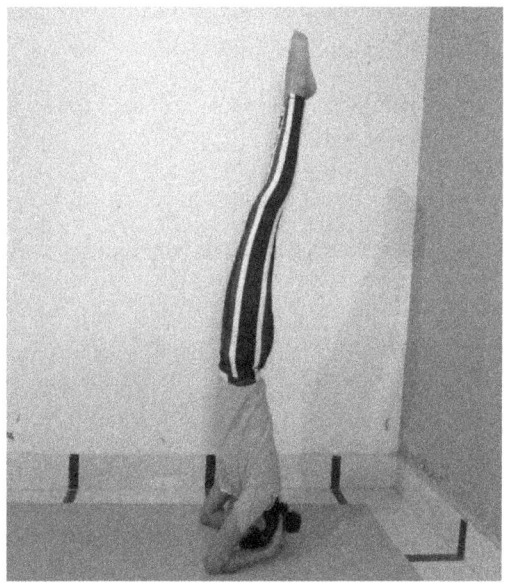

- Sit in a vajrasana, now put your elbows shoulder width apart on the ground in front of your knees and make sure your arms are horizontally out in front of you, lower yourself down onto your knees, use your arms to build your foundation, interlock the fingers of both hands into the form of a cup.
- Place your forehead on the ground, supported by your hands. Balance on your toes with your arms between your knees and your hands clasped. Slowly shift your weight forward by raising the hips, while keeping the legs still bent.
- Gradually shift your weight on your elbows and there should be a lot of pressure on your head.

- Raising your Body Straighten your legs. Extend both of your legs and raise your buttocks in the air. Keep your knees straight.
- Walk your feet towards your hands slowly lift your feet off the floor then stretch your legs upwards.
- Maintain your balance by focusing on pushing through your back, shoulder and arm into the ground.
- Maintain this pose for one minute.
- Releasing from the Pose slowly. Lower the knees back down to the chest. Place both feet on the floor. Return to your hands and knees. Bend the knees and lower your hips. Roll back into a Vajrasana posture.
- Now lower yourself into a supine position by creating a comfortable and relaxing position.
- Close your eyes and focus on your breathing.
- Then stand up and gradually stretch the whole body upward to perform Tadasana.

TITIABHASANA

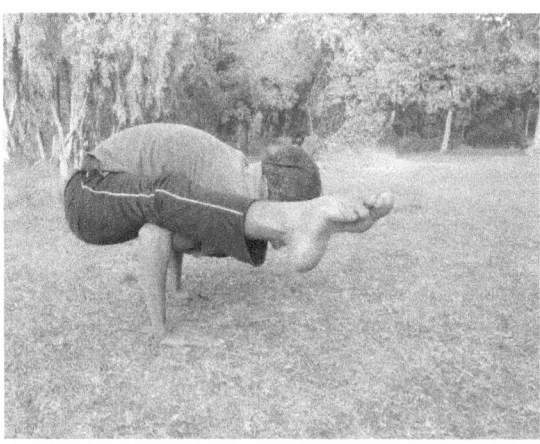

- Take your feet about 18 inches apart come into a forward band with your knees slightly bent.
- Nestle your shoulders as far under your knees as you can. You can bend your knees more if you need to. The third on the upper arms will do.

- Bring your palms flat on the floor first behind your feet.
- Bend your elbow slightly back as you would, if you were heading into chaturangadandasana.
- Begin to shift your weight back to rest on your upper arms. Let the slide back word moment lift your feet up off the floor.
- Strengthen your arm as much as possible.
- Strengthen your legs and hang your upper arm starting with your thighs.
- Flex your feet. To come out, bend your knees and tip your feet forward until they touch.

Ustrasana

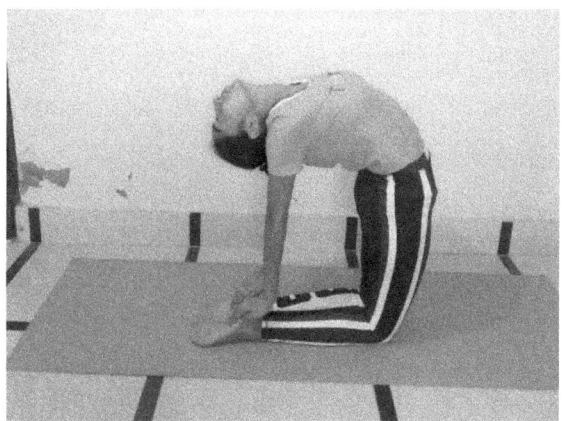

- Relax the body in the mountain taking deep breaths.
- Exhale and move your torso forward from the hips, not the waist.
- Continue to bend till your hands touch your feet take a few breaths.
- Stretch your hips and bend further.
- Place the palm of your hands by the side of your feet.
- Bring your forehead to your knees, close your eyes and relax the body.
- Take deep and slow breaths. Hold the position for a few seconds.
- As you retain the pose, gently try to stretch the spine further.

VATAYANASANA

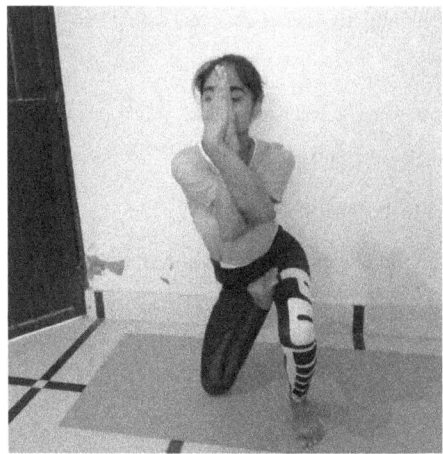

- Relax the body in a mountain pose taking deep breaths.
- Exhale and move your torso forwards from the hips, not the waist.
- Continue to bend till your hands touch your feet and take a few breaths.
- Stretch your hips and bend further (without streaming the body).
- Place the palm of your hands by the side of your feet.
- Bring your forehead to your knees. Close your eyes and relax the body.
- Take deep and slow breaths. Hold the position for a few seconds.
- As you retain the pose, gently try to stretch the spine further.

VRISCHIKASANA

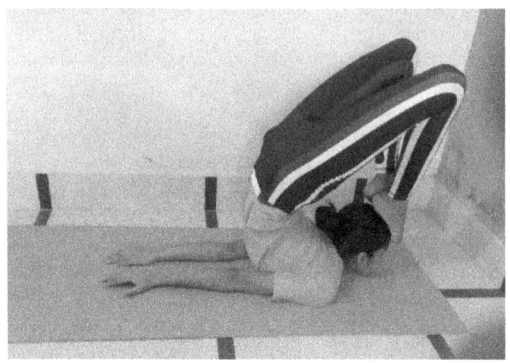

- Assume Shirshasana's ultimate position. Take a normal breath.
- Relax your entire body by bending your knees and arching your back.
- Your lower arms should be parallel to each other, and your palms should be level on the floor.
- Maintain equilibrium by shifting the weight to your forearms.
- Lower the feet to the level of the head.
- Raise your brows backwards and upwards.
- Raise your upper arms to a vertical position.
- In the ultimate stance, the heels should rest on the crown of the head.
- Your entire body should be relaxed.
- Stay in this position for as long as you want.
- Lower your legs and release into Shirshasana.

VIBHAKTA PASCHIMOTTANASANA

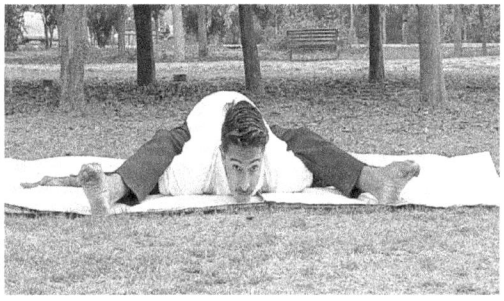

- Sit up straight and stretch your legs out in front of you. Then, with both feet pointed straight up at the ceiling, do the same.
- Make sure you're sitting tall and your spine is straight.
- Take a deep breath and stretch your arms up above your head.
- As you come down, exhale and lean forward, bringing your hands towards your feet.
- Wrapping your index fingers around your big toes is the perfect hand posture if you can reach your feet.

VAJRASANA

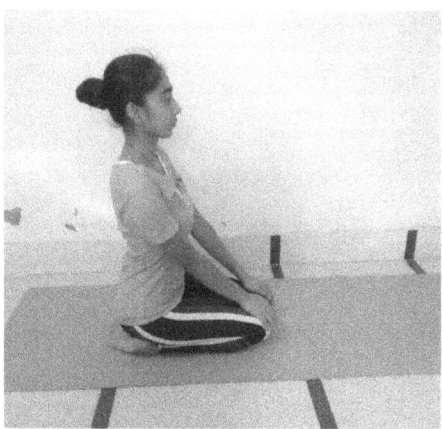

- Kneel on the floor to begin. For added comfort, consider utilizing a yoga mat.
- Bring your knees and ankles together and line up your feet with your legs. Your big toes should touch, and the bottoms of your feet should face upward.
- As you sit back on your legs, exhale. Your thighs will rest on your calves, while your buttocks will rest on your heels.
- Place your hands on your thighs and gently move your pelvis back and forth until you're comfortable.
- Slowly inhale and exhale while positioning yourself to sit up straight by straightening your spine. Pull your body upward with your head and your tailbone toward the floor.
- Straighten your neck so that your chin is parallel to the floor and you may look forward. Place your hands palms down on your thighs and relax your arms.

PRANAYAMAS AND KRIYAS:

Important instruction common to all pranayamas:

- Pranayam should be performed on an empty stomach with a five-hour break between meals and practice.
- Choosing the places for Pranayama should be full of air and relaxing. Pranayama should not be done when it is too chilly or too hot. Sit comfortably in any

contemplative asana, such as Padmasana, Ardha Padmasana, Siddhasana, or Sukhasana.

- The goal of a Yoga practitioner is to achieve God, so meditate on Him and cease thinking about everything else.
- Beginners should begin with three rounds of Pranayam and gradually increase the number of rounds as they gain experience.
- Breathe easily during pranayam; otherwise, it will be damaging to us, particularly to our neurological system. So if you're feeling perplexed, gradually release the pranayama as directed.
- Beginners who are unable to conduct Pranayama continuously might take two or three regular breaths in between each cycle of pranayama.
- Pranayama should only be practiced under the supervision of a professional if you have heart disease or hypertension.

KRIYAS

- Neti is one of the six shatkarma cleansing techniques.
- Dhauti is a procedure for cleansing the upper stomach.
- Neti-Nasal cleansing procedure known as neti.
- Nauli-Massages the abdominal organs.
- Basti-The cleansing of the big intestine is known as basti.
- Kapalbhati- A breathing method in which the forehead shines.
- Trataka - A purifying exercise for the eyes and muscles.

JAL NETI

Jal Neti is a technique utilized by yogis to keep disease-free and, more importantly, to utilize their breath effectively in their yoga activities. Jal Neti is nose hygiene in the same way as brushing your teeth is dental hygiene. Water is used to purify and clear the nasal passageway, which runs from the nostrils to the throat. In Jal Neti salty lukewarm water is used to clear nasal and respiratory congestion and obstructions. Jal Neti aids in the prevention of numerous ailments as well as the smooth passage of air via the nostrils.

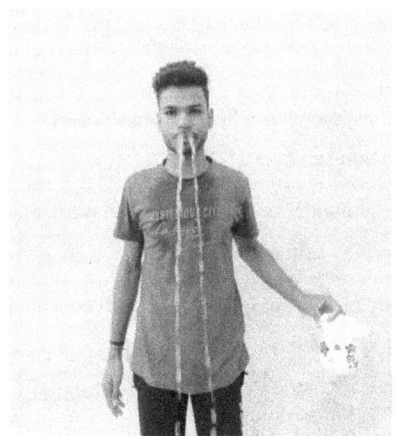

Steps

- To begin, choose a neti pot that has a nozzle that can easily be placed into the nostril.
- In half a litre of lukewarm water, dissolve one teaspoon of salt.
- Fill the neti pot halfway with this water.
- To begin, sit in Kagasana with a 1-foot gap between your legs.
- From your lower back, lean forward.
- Tilt your head to the side of the nostril that is the most active at the time.
- Insert the pot's nozzle into the nostril that is active at the time.
- Throughout the neti process, keep your mouth open and try to breathe through it.
- Allow water to enter through one nostril and exit through the other.
- Place the Neti pot down after using half of the water and clear your nostril.
- The same should be done on the other side.
- Exhale forcefully from both nostrils in all directions (left and right, top and bottom) after finishing on both sides.

SUTRA NETI

Sutra is a Sanskrit phrase that literally means "thread," while Neti refers to "nasal cleaning." Sutra neti is a method of cleaning the nasal passages with a cotton thread or rubber catheter. Depending on the type of thread used, it's also known as Thread Neti or Rubber Neti.

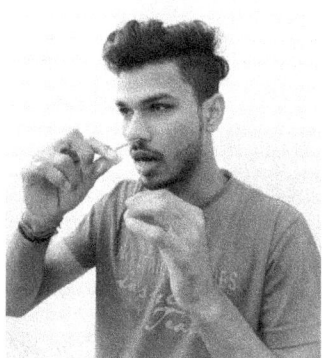

- Take a cable made of thread dipped in beeswax or a catheter made of rubber in place of the thread. Rinse the cord with warm water or specific oils or drugs before properly drying it.
- Slowly and gently insert the thread into one of the nostrils. Keep the cable pointing backwards in your throat.
- Using your index and middle fingers, reach into your mouth and grab the cable at the back of the throat.
- Reach the thread at the back of the throat and gently pull it out of the mouth.
- With both hands, hold both ends of the string and move it back and forth two or three times.
- Rep the procedure with the other nostril.
- Sutra neti can be performed by transferring the string from one nostril to the other once the previous process is understood.

PRANAYAMA:

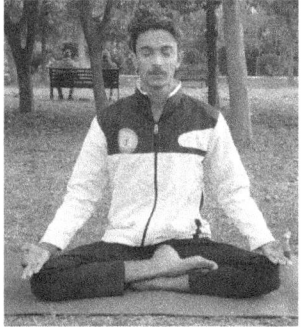

BHRAMARI PRANAYAM

- Sit comfortably in any contemplative asana, such as Padmasana, Ardha Padmasana, Siddhasana, or Sukhasana, in a light, open space.
- Close your eyes for a few moments and notice the sensations in your body. Feel the inner peace.
- Please place your thumb on the tragus of the ear and press it down so that the external auditory meatus of the ears is closed.
- Place your index finger right above the brows on the forehead.
- Place your middle finger on your closed eyes and the tip of your finger on the caruncle of your eyes without putting any pressure on them.
- On the nasofacial angle, place your fourth and fifth fingers.
- Now progressively descend towards hell while creating a loud bee-like buzzing sound from the throat.
- Place your index finger right above the brows on the forehead.
- Place your middle finger on your closed eyes and the tip of your finger on the caruncle of your eyes without putting any pressure on them.
- On the nasofacial angle, place your fourth and fifth fingers.
- Now progressively descend towards hell while creating a loud bee-like buzzing sound from the throat.

KAPALBHATI PRANAYAMAS

- Sit in a comfortable position with your spine straight. Put your hands on your knees, palms facing the sky.
- Take a deep breath in and exhale slowly.
- Pull your navel back towards your spine as you exhale. Do as much as you are able to comfortably. You can feel the abdominal muscles contract by placing your right hand on the stomach.
- The breath pours into your lungs effortlessly as you relax your navel and abdomen.

- To finish one round of Kapal Bhati, take 20 such breaths.
- Kapal Bhati's exhale is energetic and strong. So simply let out a sigh of relief.
- Don't be concerned about inhaling. Inhalation will occur automatically as soon as your abdominal muscles relax.
- Maintain your focus on exhaling.
- Relax with your eyes closed after completing the round and pay attention to the sensations in your body.
- Two additional rounds of Kapal Bhati are required.

NADISHODHAN PRANAYAMA

- Sit back in your chair, calm and with a soft smile on your face. Maintain a relaxed shoulder and a straight spine.
- Place your left hand on the back of your left knee. The palm of your hand should be open to the sky or in a chin posture.
- Between your brows, place your middle and index fingers. Keep your thumb on the right side of your nostril and your little and ring fingers on the left. The ring and little fingers will be used to open and close the left nostril. In addition, the thumb is used to clean the right nostril.
- Exhale through your left nose while pressing your thumb against your right nostril.
- After you've breathed through your left nostril, softly press the left portion of the nostril with your little and index fingers.
- Exhale from the right side by letting go of the thumb on that side.
- Inhale via your right nostril and exhale through your left. The first round of Pranayama is now complete.
- Breathe through alternate nostrils in the same way.

SURYA NAMASKARA

The Sanskrit word surya refers to the sun and namaskara means 'greeting'. In yoga the sun is represented by the pingala or Surya Nadi, a pranic channel containing vital, life-giving energy. It's perfect Sadhana, a spiritual act, itself includes the Asana, Pranayama, mantra and meditation techniques. Surya namaskar is a beautiful combination of 12 yogic asanas. It was good cardiovascular. It improves blood circulation in our body. It is a good physical practice as well as calms your mind, removes stress and is helpful to reduce anxiety also. It is a very good practice for mind and energy body and spiritual body as well. While performing Surya namaskar your breathing should be in flow.

Ideal time for Surya namaskar -You can do it at the sunrise.

Step-1 (Pranamasana)

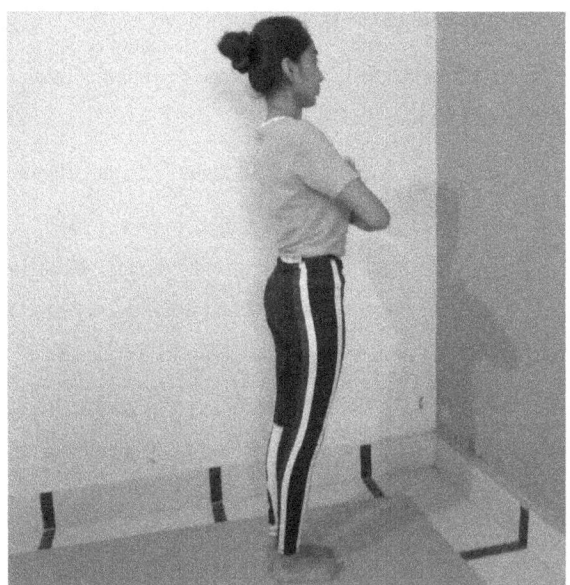

- Standing in a natural position facing the sun.
- Shoulders should be relaxed.
- Firstly, Inhale then exhale.
- Keep your feet together and palm joint in a prayer or namaskar pose at your heart centre.
- Relax your whole body.
- Take a deep breath to regulate your breathing.

Step-2 (Hastottanasana)

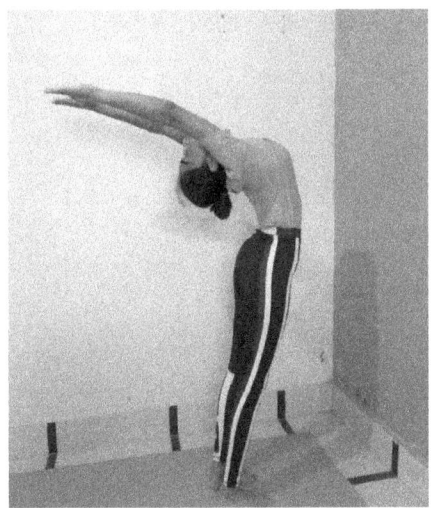

- Inhale, raise your arms above your head in upward salute.
- Shoulders are relaxed.
- Namaskar tilts slightly backward arching.
- Your back looks at your hands.
- Keep your lower body straight as much as possible.

Step-3 (Hastapadasana)

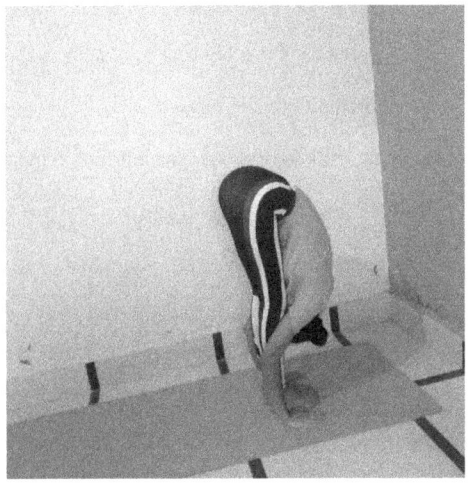

- Exhale slowly, Bend forward,
- Placing your palms on either side or in front of your feet.
- Your forehead touching your knees.
- Do not strain.
- Your ankle, knee and hip lie in one line.
- Your weight on your heels and toes equally.

Step-4 (Ashwa Sanchalanasana)

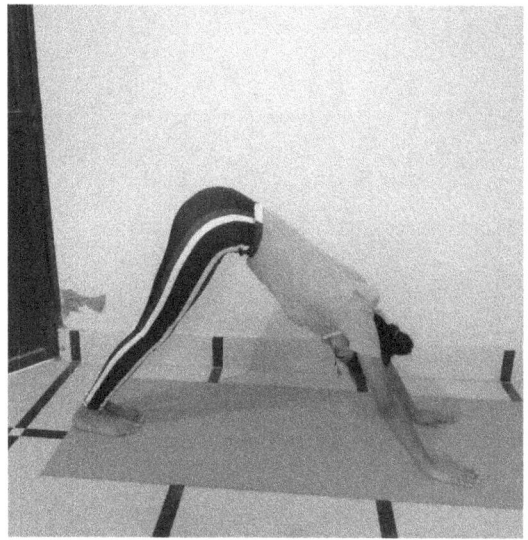

- Inhale and take your right leg back in a big backward step.
- Right knee and flat foot on the floor and relaxed.
- At the same time bend the left knee but keep the left foot in the same position.
- Keep your hands firmly in place.
- Your left foot must be over your ankle between your hands.
- In the final position, the weight of the body should be supported on two hands, the left foot and the right knee and toes of the right foot.
- Tilt your head up with slow exhalation.

Step-5 (Dandasana)

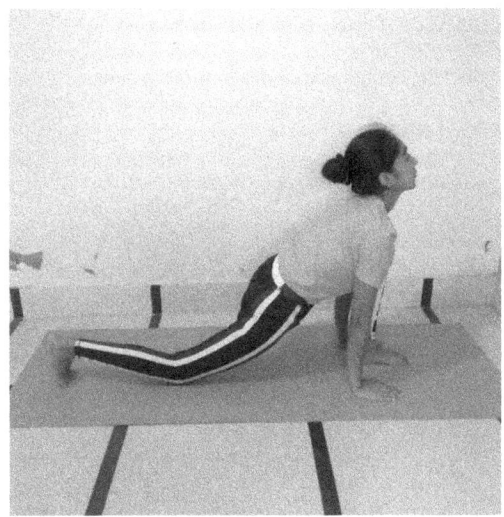

- Exhale, move your left foot back to where your right foot is.
- Your whole body is in one line.
- Lower the head so that it lies between the two arms.
- Keep your arms straight.
- Raise your hip. Bring your head close to the floor.
- Try to keep the heels in contact with the ground in this pose.
- Inhale deeply your body should form an inverted v do not bend your knee.

Step-6 (Ashtanga Namaskar)

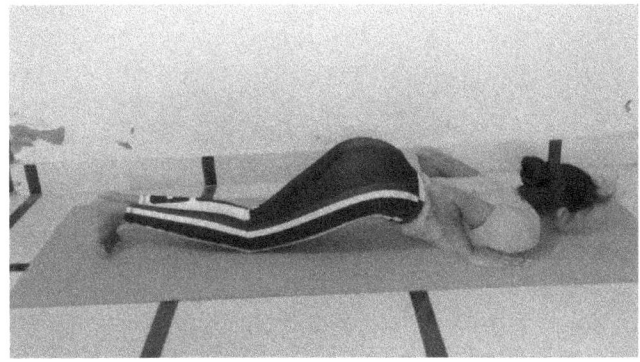

- Exhale and lower the body to the floor.
- Only the forehead, chest, hands and feet touch the floor.
- The hip and abdomen should raise slightly off the ground.
- Elbow should be close to the body.

Step-7 (Bhujangasana)

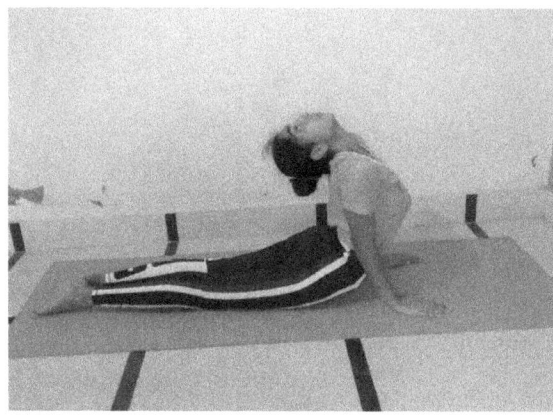

- Inhale, lift your chest into the cobra pose.
- Bend the head backward.
- And keep your arm straight and in place.
- Torso till belly button upward.
- Shoulders are relaxed.

Step-8 (Adho Mukha Svanasana)

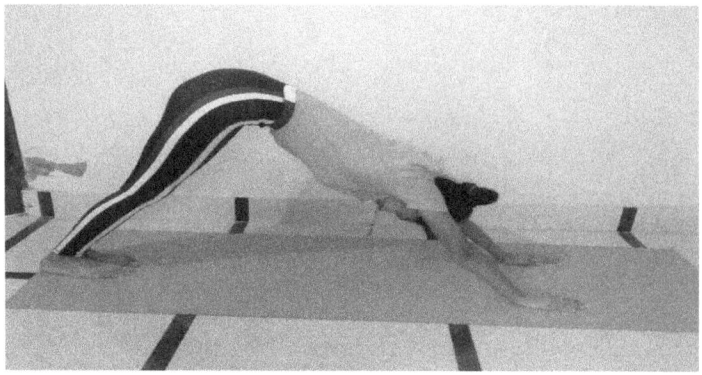

- This stage is a repeat of position 5.
- Exhale and tuck your toes under.
- Lift your whole body.
- Slowly raise your hips to come back to the inverted V.
- From the back position assume the mountain pose.
- Do not bend your knees.

Step-9 (Ashwa Sanchalanasana)

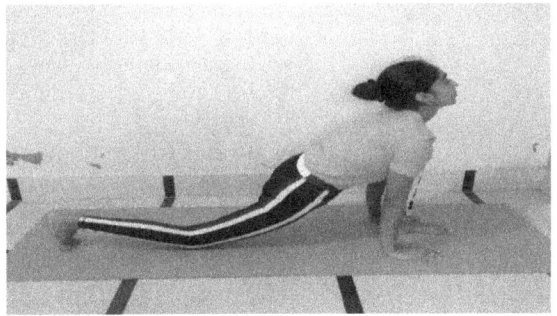

- This stage is same as position 4
- Inhale and move your right leg forward.
- Your left knee and foot are on the floor in a relaxed position.
- Placing your right foot between your hands.
- Tilt your head up.

Step-10 (Hasta Padasana)

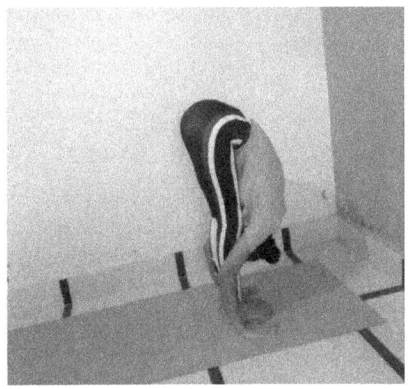

- This stage is a repeat of position 3.
- Exhale slowly and rise bringing your left foot forward to where your right foot is,
- See that the hands and leg are in line and your head touches the knees.
- do not strain if you are unable to touch the knee but do not bend the legs.

Step-11 (Hasta Uttanasana)

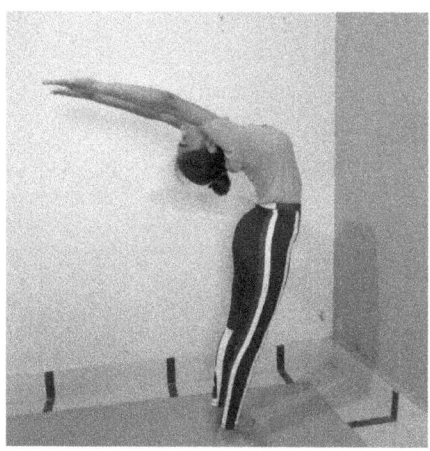

- This stage is the same as position 2.
- Inhale and raise your arm above your head in the upward salute pose.
- Tilt slightly backward, arching your back-stand firm in place.

Step-12

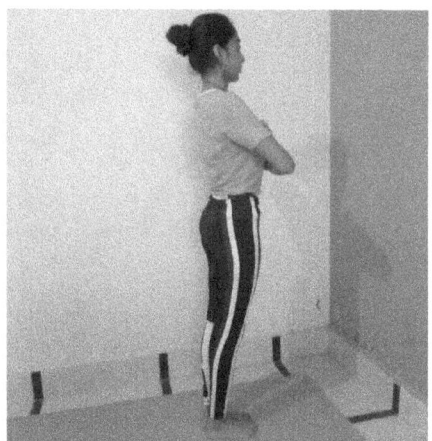

- This is a final pose and is the same as position 1. Exhale and slowly bring down your hands to your chest in the prayer pose.
- Relax the whole body.

3.5 STATISTICAL TECHNIQUES USED

The statistical analysis was carried out using IBM SPSS (Statistical Package for Social Sciences) statistical version 20. All quantitative variables were estimated using measures of central location (mean and median) and measures of dispersion (standard deviation). Normality of data was checked by Skewness and Kurtosis. For normality distributed data, Mean was compared with respect to One-way ANOVA (for more than two groups) and after One-way ANOVA significant using Post Hoc Least Significant Difference Test (LSD) for multiple comparison. For normality distributed data, Mean was compared at pre and post using Dependent t-test. For normality distributed data, Pearson Correlation Method was used for relationship between parameters. All statistical tests were seen at two-tailed levels of significance ($p \leq 0.01$ and $p \leq 0.05$). ANOVA and t-test were used to analyze the data collected from experimental groups before and after Yoga training of University players through SPSS software. Based on these tools, procedures, methods and statistical calculations, the analysis of the results are shown in the next chapter.

CHAPTER 4

ANALYSIS AND INTERPRETATION OF DATA

In this chapter researchers described about the statistics of various variables such as results of the study. Descriptive statistics involved mean, standard deviation. Mean is the measure of Central tendency standard deviation defines the measure of dispersion screen s is the measure of symmetry.

4.1 DESCRIPTIVE STATISTICS FOR DIFFERENT VARIABLES

Table 4.1.1: Descriptive statistics of PGI memory scale (PGI) and problem-solving ability test (PSAT) for pre and post of yoga camp for players from Chaudhary Devi Lal University (CDLU), Sirsa

	PGI PRE	PSAT PRE	PGI POST	PSAT POST
N	25	25	25	25
Mean	60.32	7.92	68.96	10.88
Std. Deviation	5.68	1.98	4.24	2.01

The above table depicts the descriptive statistics of various variables such as results of PGI memory scale and PSAT for players from Chaudhary Devi Lal University (CDLU), Sirsa before and after performing yogasanas. Descriptive statistics involved mean, standard deviation. Mean is the measure of central tendency, standard deviation defines the measure of dispersion.

As shown in the above table, total numbers of respondents were 25, for PGI pre, the mean value was 60.385 with standard deviation of 5.579. For PSAT pre, the mean was 7.923 and standard deviation was 1.937. After attending the yoga camp and performing yogasanas, the mean for results of the PGI memory scale test (PGI post) increased to 69.077 with standard deviation 4.195. Similarly, there was an increase in PSAT results after performing yogasanas (PSAT post) with mean 10.962, standard deviation 2.010.

Table 4.1.2: Descriptive statistics of PGI memory scale (PGI) and problem-solving ability test (PSAT) for pre and post of yoga camp for players from Chaudhary Ranbir Singh University (CRSU), Jind

	PGI PRE	PSAT PRE	PGI POST	PSAT POST
N	25	25	25	25
Mean	60.12	10.24	68.60	12.76
Std. Deviation	6.41	3.42	5.06	2.45

The above table depicts the descriptive statistics of variables PGI memory scale and PSAT for players from Chaudhary Ranbir Singh University (CRSU), Jind before and after attending the yoga camp. Granting the above table, total number of players/respondents were 25, for PGI pre, the mean value was 60.12 with standard deviation of 6.41. For PSAT pre, the mean was 10.24 and standard deviation was 3.42. After performing yogasanas, the mean for the results of PGI memory scale test (PGI post) increased to 68.60 with standard deviation 5.06. Likewise, there was an increase in PSAT results after attending the yoga camp and performing yogasanas (PSAT post) with mean 12.76, standard deviation 2.45.

Table 4.1.3: Descriptive statistics of PGI memory scale (PGI) and problem-solving ability test (PSAT) for pre and post of yoga camp for players from Kurukshetra University, Kurukshetra (KUK)

	PGI PRE	PSAT PRE	PGI POST	PSAT POST
N	25	25	25	25
Mean	65.20	8.80	73.36	13.48
Std. Deviation	4.69	2.66	3.93	2.60

The above table depicts the descriptive statistics of various variables such as results of PGI memory scale and PSAT for players from Kurukshetra University, Kurukshetra (KUK), before and after performing yogasanas. As shown in the above table, total numbers of respondents were 25, for PGI pre, the mean value was 65.20 with standard deviation of 4.69. For PSAT pre, the mean was 8.80 and standard deviation was 2.66. After attending the yoga camp and performing yogasanas, the mean for results of PGI memory scale test (PGI post) increased to 73.36 with standard deviation 3.93. Similarly, there was an increase in results of PSAT after performing yogasanas (PSAT post) with mean 13.48, standard deviation 2.60.

Table 4.1.4: Descriptive statistics of PGI memory scale (PGI) and problem-solving ability test (PSAT) for pre and post of yoga camp for players from Maharshi Dayanand University (MDU), Rohtak

	PGI PRE	PSAT PRE	PGI POST	PSAT POST
N	25	25	25	25
Mean	62.16	9.08	71.44	12.96
Std. Deviation	8.19	2.55	4.71	1.90

The above table depicts the descriptive statistics of variables PGI memory scale and PSAT for players from Maharshi Dayanand University (MDU), Rohtak before and after attending the yoga camp. As shown by the figures in the above table, total number of players/respondents was 25, for PGI pre, i.e. results for PGI memory scale test before attending the yoga camp, the mean value was 62.16 with standard deviation of 9.08. For PSAT pre, i.e. results for problem-solving ability test before attending the yoga camp, the mean was 9.08 and standard deviation was 2.55. After performing yogasanas, the mean for results of PGI memory scale test (PGI post) increased to 71.44 with standard deviation 4.71. Likewise, there was an increase in PSAT results after attending the yoga camp and performing yogasanas (PSAT post) with mean 12.96, standard deviation 1.90.

Table 4.1.5: Descriptive statistics of subtests of PGI memory scale (PGI) before attending the yoga camp for players from Chaudhary Devi Lal University (CDLU), Sirsa

	N	Mean	Std. Deviation
Remote Memory	25	5.80	0.82
Recent Memory	25	5.88	0.83
Mental Balance	25	6.80	1.35
Attention and Concentration	25	4.96	1.34
Delayed Recall	25	9.52	1.96
Immediate Recall	25	7.12	2.51
Retention for Similar Pairs	25	6.16	0.90
Retention for Dissimilar Pairs	25	4.88	0.93
Visual Retention	25	4.68	0.95
Recognition	25	4.52	0.87

The above table depicts the descriptive statistics of the results of ten subtests of PGI memory scale test such as, remote memory, recent memory, mental balance, attention and concentration, delayed recall, immediate recall, retention for similar pairs, retention for dissimilar pairs, visual retention, and recognition, of players from Chaudhary Devi Lal University (CDLU), Sirsa before attending the yoga camp. The descriptive statistics include mean, standard deviation. For remote memory test, the mean was 5.80 with standard deviation 0.82. For recent memory test, mean was 5.88, standard deviation was 0.83. Mental balance test has mean value of 6.80 with standard deviation of 1.35. For attention and concentration test, the mean value was 4.96, and standard deviation was 1.35. For delayed recall test, the mean was 9.52 with standard deviation 1.96. For immediate recall test, mean was 7.12, and standard deviation was 2.51. Retention for similar pairs test has mean value of 6.16 with standard deviation of 0.90. For retention for dissimilar pairs test, the mean value was 4.88, and standard deviation was 0.93. For visual retention test, the mean was 4.68 with standard deviation 0.95. And, for recognition test, mean was 4.52, and standard deviation was 0.87.

Table 4.1.6: Descriptive statistics of subtests of PGI memory scale (PGI) after attending the yoga camp for players from Chaudhary Devi Lal University (CDLU), Sirsa

	N	Mean	Std. Deviation
Remote Memory	25	6.32	0.75
Recent Memory	25	6.36	0.76
Mental Balance	25	7.08	1.22
Attention and Concentration	25	4.96	1.17
Delayed Recall	25	9.92	1.26
Immediate Recall	25	9.28	2.69
Retention for Similar Pairs	25	5.72	0.68
Retention for Dissimilar Pairs	25	10.48	2.24
Visual Retention	25	4.84	0.85
Recognition	25	4.00	0.87

The above table explains the descriptive statistics of the results of ten subtests of PGI memory scale test such as, remote memory, recent memory, mental balance, attention and concentration, delayed recall, immediate recall, retention for similar pairs, retention for dissimilar pairs, visual retention, and recognition, of players from Chaudhary Devi Lal University (CDLU), Sirsa after attending the yoga camp. For remote memory test, the mean was 6.32 with standard deviation 0.75. For recent memory test, mean was 6.36, and standard deviation was 0.76. Mental balance test has mean value of 7.08 with standard deviation of 1.22. For attention and concentration test, the mean value was 4.96, standard deviation was 1.17. For delayed recall test, the mean was 9.92 with standard deviation 1.26. For immediate recall test, mean was 9.28, and standard deviation was 2.69. Retention for similar pairs test has mean value of 5.72 with standard deviation of 0.68. For retention for dissimilar pairs test, the mean value was 10.48, and standard deviation was 2.24. For visual retention test, the mean was 4.84 with standard deviation 0.85. And, for recognition test, mean was 4.00, standard deviation was 0.87.

Table 4.1.7: Descriptive statistics of subtests of PGI memory scale (PGI) before attending the yoga camp for players from Chaudhary Ranbir Singh University (CRSU), Jind

	N	Mean	Std. Deviation
Remote Memory	25	5.64	0.99
Recent Memory	25	5.68	1.03
Mental Balance	25	7.16	0.94
Attention and Concentration	25	4.84	1.91
Delayed Recall	25	9.60	1.41
Immediate Recall	25	7.40	1.78
Retention for Similar Pairs	25	6.04	1.24
Retention for Dissimilar Pairs	25	4.72	0.84
Visual Retention	25	4.52	1.12
Recognition	25	4.52	1.08

The above table depicts the descriptive statistics of the results of ten subtests of PGI memory scale test such as, remote memory, recent memory, mental balance, attention and concentration, delayed recall, immediate recall, retention for similar pairs, retention for dissimilar pairs, visual retention, and recognition, of players from Chaudhary Ranbir Singh University (CRSU), Jind before attending the yoga camp.

The descriptive statistics include mean, standard deviation, skewness, and kurtosis. For remote memory test, the mean was 5.64 with standard deviation 0.99. For recent memory test, mean was 5.68, standard deviation was 1.03. Mental balance test has mean value of 7.16 with standard deviation of 0.94. For attention and concentration test, the mean value was 4.84, and standard deviation was 1.91. For delayed recall test, the mean was 9.60 with standard deviation 1.41. For immediate recall test, mean was 7.40, and standard deviation was 1.78. Retention for similar pairs test has mean value of 6.04 with standard deviation of 1.24. For retention for dissimilar pairs test, the mean value was 4.72, and standard deviation was 0.84. For visual retention test, the mean was 4.52 with standard deviation 1.12. And, for recognition test, mean was 4.52, and standard deviation was 1.08.

Table 4.1.8: Descriptive statistics of subtests of PGI memory scale (PGI) after attending the yoga camp for players from Chaudhary Ranbir Singh University (CRSU), Jind

	N	Mean	Std. Deviation
Remote Memory	25	6.16	0.90
Recent Memory	25	6.16	0.90
Mental Balance	25	6.52	1.45
Attention and Concentration	25	4.80	1.12
Delayed Recall	25	9.44	1.58
Immediate Recall	25	10.12	2.44
Retention for Similar Pairs	25	5.48	1.00
Retention for Dissimilar Pairs	25	10.56	1.69
Visual Retention	25	5.04	0.84
Recognition	25	4.32	1.07

The above table represents the descriptive statistics of the results of ten subtests of PGI memory scale test such as, remote memory, recent memory, mental balance, attention and concentration, delayed recall, immediate recall, retention for similar pairs, retention for dissimilar pairs, visual retention, and recognition, of players from Chaudhary Ranbir Singh University (CRSU), Jind after attending the yoga camp. For remote memory test, the mean was 6.16 with standard deviation 0.90. For recent memory test, mean was 6.16, and standard deviation was 0.90. Mental balance test has mean value of 6.52 with standard deviation of 1.45. For attention and concentration test, the mean value was 4.80, and standard deviation was 1.12. For delayed recall test, the mean was 9.44 with standard deviation 1.58. For immediate recall test, mean was 10.12, and standard deviation was 2.44. Retention for similar pairs test has mean value of 5.48 with standard deviation of 1.00. For retention for dissimilar pairs test, the mean value was 10.56, and standard deviation was 1.69. For visual retention test, the mean was 5.04 with standard deviation 0.84. And, for recognition test, mean was 4.32, standard deviation was 1.07.

Table 4.1.9: Descriptive statistics of subtests of PGI memory scale (PGI) before attending the yoga camp for players from Kurukshetra University, Kurukshetra (KUK)

	N	Mean	Std. Deviation
Remote Memory	25	6.08	1.12
Recent Memory	25	6.12	1.13
Mental Balance	25	7.68	1.25
Attention and Concentration	25	4.48	1.50
Delayed Recall	25	9.36	1.66
Immediate Recall	25	7.04	2.89
Retention for Similar Pairs	25	6.48	1.05
Retention for Dissimilar Pairs	25	6.20	1.63
Visual Retention	25	6.04	1.40
Recognition	25	5.72	1.46

The above table exhibits the descriptive statistics of the results of ten subtests of PGI memory scale test such as, remote memory, recent memory, mental balance, attention and concentration, delayed recall, immediate recall, retention for similar pairs, retention for dissimilar pairs, visual retention, and recognition, of players from Kurukshetra University, Kurukshetra (KUK) before attending the yoga camp. The descriptive statistics include mean, standard deviation, skewness, and kurtosis. For remote memory test, the mean was 6.08 with standard deviation 1.12. For recent memory test, mean was 6.12, and standard deviation was 1.13. Mental balance test has mean value of 7.68 with standard deviation of 1.25. For attention and concentration test, the mean value was 4.48, and standard deviation was 1.50. For delayed recall test, the mean was 9.36 with standard deviation 1.66. For immediate recall test, mean was 7.04, and standard deviation was 2.89. Retention for similar pairs test has mean value of 6.48 with standard deviation of 1.05. For retention for dissimilar pairs test, the mean value was 6.20, and standard deviation was 1.63. For visual retention test, the mean was 6.04 with standard deviation 1.40. And, for recognition test, mean was 5.72, and standard deviation was 1.46.

Table 4.1.10: Descriptive statistics of subtests of PGI memory scale (PGI) after attending the yoga camp for players from Kurukshetra University, Kurukshetra (KUK)

	N	Mean	Std. Deviation
Remote Memory	25	6.76	0.83
Recent Memory	25	6.68	0.80
Mental Balance	25	8.28	1.43
Attention and Concentration	25	5.32	1.46
Delayed Recall	25	10.44	1.04
Immediate Recall	25	10.16	2.23
Retention for Similar Pairs	25	6.20	0.87
Retention for Dissimilar Pairs	25	8.96	2.59
Visual Retention	25	5.64	0.95
Recognition	25	4.92	1.15

The above table shows the descriptive statistics of the results of ten subtests of PGI memory scale test such as, remote memory, recent memory, mental balance, attention and concentration, delayed recall, immediate recall, retention for similar pairs, retention for dissimilar pairs, visual retention, and recognition, of players from Kurukshetra University, Kurukshetra (KUK) after attending the yoga camp. For remote memory test, the mean was 6.76 with standard deviation 0.83. For recent memory test, mean was 6.68, and standard deviation was 0.80. Mental balance test has mean value of 8.28 with standard deviation of 1.43. For attention and concentration test, the mean value was 5.32, and standard deviation was 1.46. For delayed recall test, the mean was 10.44 with standard deviation 1.04. For immediate recall test, mean was 10.16, standard deviation was 2.23. Retention for similar pairs test has mean value of 6.20 with standard deviation of 0.87. For retention for dissimilar pairs test, the mean value was 8.96, and standard deviation was 2.59. For visual retention test, the mean was 5.64 with standard deviation 0.95. And, for recognition test, mean was 4.92, and standard deviation was 1.15.

Table 4.1.11: Descriptive statistics of subtests of PGI memory scale (PGI) before attending the yoga camp for players from Maharshi Dayanand University (MDU), Rohtak

	N	Mean	Std. Deviation
Remote Memory	25	7.00	1.08
Recent Memory	25	5.20	1.38
Mental Balance	25	8.28	1.62
Attention and Concentration	25	7.32	2.66
Delayed Recall	25	5.52	1.36
Immediate Recall	25	11.36	2.38
Retention for Similar Pairs	25	4.68	1.49
Retention for Dissimilar Pairs	25	4.36	1.41
Visual Retention	25	4.60	1.68
Recognition	25	3.84	1.21

The above table explains the descriptive statistics of the results of ten subtests of PGI memory scale test such as, remote memory, recent memory, mental balance, attention and concentration, delayed recall, immediate recall, retention for similar pairs, retention for dissimilar pairs, visual retention, and recognition, of players from Maharshi Dayanand University (MDU), Rohtak before attending the yoga camp. The descriptive statistics include mean, standard deviation, skewness, and kurtosis. For remote memory test, the mean was 7.00 with standard deviation 1.08. For recent memory test, mean was 5.20, and standard deviation was 1.38. Mental balance test has mean value of 8.28 with standard deviation of 1.62. For attention and concentration test, the mean value was 7.32, and standard deviation was 2.66. For delayed recall test, the mean was 5.52 with standard deviation 1.36. For immediate recall test, mean was 11.36, and standard deviation was 2.38. Retention for similar pairs test has mean value of 4.36 with standard deviation of 1.49. For retention for dissimilar pairs test, the mean value was 4.36, and standard deviation was 1.41. For visual retention test, the mean was 4.60 with standard deviation 1.68. And, for recognition test, mean was 3.84, and standard deviation was 1.21.

Table 4.1.12: Descriptive statistics of subtests of PGI memory scale (PGI) after attending the yoga camp for players from Maharshi Dayanand University (MDU), Rohtak

	N	Mean	Std. Deviation
Remote Memory	25	6.56	0.77
Recent Memory	25	6.48	0.71
Mental Balance	25	8.20	1.00
Attention and Concentration	25	5.12	0.78
Delayed Recall	25	9.68	1.55
Immediate Recall	25	9.84	2.19
Retention for Similar Pairs	25	5.60	1.08
Retention for Dissimilar Pairs	25	9.88	2.54
Visual Retention	25	5.56	1.12
Recognition	25	4.52	0.92

The above table depicts the descriptive statistics of the results of ten subtests of PGI memory scale test such as, remote memory, recent memory, mental balance, attention and concentration, delayed recall, immediate recall, retention for similar pairs, retention for dissimilar pairs, visual retention, and recognition, of players from Maharshi Dayanand University (MDU), Rohtak after attending the yoga camp. For remote memory test, the mean was 6.56 with standard deviation 0.77. For recent memory test, mean was 6.48, and standard deviation was 0.71. Mental balance test has mean value of 8.20 with standard deviation of 1.00. For attention and concentration test, the mean value was 5.12, and standard deviation was 0.78. For delayed recall test, the mean was 9.68 with standard deviation 1.55. For immediate recall test, mean was 9.84, and standard deviation was 2.19. Retention for similar pairs test has mean value of 5.60 with standard deviation of 1.08. For retention for dissimilar pairs test, the mean value was 9.88, and standard deviation was 2.54. For visual retention test, the mean was 5.56 with standard deviation 1.12. And, for recognition test, mean was 4.52, and standard deviation was 0.92.

Table 4.1.13: Descriptive statistics of subtests of PGI memory scale (PGI) before attending the yoga camp for all players

	N	Mean	Std. Deviation
Remote Memory	100	6.13	1.13
Recent Memory	100	5.72	1.15
Mental Balance	100	7.48	1.41
Attention and Concentration	100	5.40	2.20
Delayed Recall	100	8.50	2.35
Immediate Recall	100	8.23	3.00
Retention for Similar Pairs	100	5.84	1.36
Retention for Dissimilar Pairs	100	5.04	1.41
Visual Retention	100	4.96	1.44
Recognition	100	4.65	1.34

The above table represents the descriptive statistics of the results of ten subtests of PGI memory scale test such as, remote memory, recent memory, mental balance, attention and concentration, delayed recall, immediate recall, retention for similar pairs, retention for dissimilar pairs, visual retention, and recognition, of players irrespective of their universities, before attending the yoga camp. The total number of respondents were 100. For remote memory test, the mean was 6.13 with standard deviation 1.13. For recent memory test, mean was 5.72, and standard deviation was 1.15. Mental balance test has mean value of 7.48 with standard deviation of 1.41. For attention and concentration test, the mean value was 5.40, and standard deviation was 2.20. For delayed recall test, the mean was 8.50 with standard deviation 2.35. For immediate recall test, mean was 8.23, and standard deviation was 3.00. Retention for similar pairs test has mean value of 5.84 with standard deviation of 1.36. For retention for dissimilar pairs test, the mean value was 5.04, and standard deviation was 1.41. For visual retention test, the mean was 4.96 with standard deviation 1.44. And, for recognition test, mean was 4.65, and standard deviation was 1.34.

Table 4.1.14: Descriptive statistics of subtests of PGI memory scale (PGI) after attending the yoga camp for all players

	N	Mean	Std. Deviation
Remote Memory	100	6.45	0.83
Recent Memory	100	6.42	0.81
Mental Balance	100	7.52	1.47
Attention and Concentration	100	5.05	1.16
Delayed Recall	100	9.87	1.40
Immediate Recall	100	9.85	2.38
Retention for Similar Pairs	100	5.75	0.95
Retention for Dissimilar Pairs	100	9.97	2.35
Visual Retention	100	5.27	0.99
Recognition	100	4.44	1.05

The above table explains the descriptive statistics of the results of ten subtests of PGI memory scale test such as, remote memory, recent memory, mental balance, attention and concentration, delayed recall, immediate recall, retention for similar pairs, retention for dissimilar pairs, visual retention, and recognition, of players irrespective of their universities, after attending the yoga camp. For remote memory test, the mean was 6.45 with standard deviation 0.83. For recent memory test, mean was 6.42, and standard deviation was 0.81. Mental balance test has mean value of 7.52 with standard deviation of 1.47. For attention and concentration test, the mean value was 5.05, and standard deviation was 1.16. For delayed recall test, the mean was 9.87 with standard deviation 1.40. For immediate recall test, meanwas 9.85, and standard deviation was 2.38. Retention for similar pairs test has mean value of 5.75 with standard deviation of 0.95. For retention for dissimilar pairs test, the mean value was9.97, standard deviation was 2.35. For visual retention test, the mean was 5.27 with standard deviation 0.99. And, for recognition test, mean was 4.44, and standard deviation was 1.05.

OBJECTIVE 1

THE EFFECT OF THE YOGA ON MEMORY OF PLAYERS

Hypotheses involved:

1: There will be no significant difference of yoga on memory of players.

1.a.: There will be no significant difference of yoga on remote memory of players.

1.b.: There will be no significant difference of yoga on recent memory of players.

1.c.: There will be no significant difference of yoga on mental balance of players.

1.d.: There will be no significant difference of yoga on attention and concentration of players.

1.e.: There will be no significant difference of yoga on delayed recall of players.

1.f.: There will be no significant difference of yoga on immediate recall of players.

1.g.: There will be no significant difference of yoga on retention for similar pairs of players.

1.h.: There will be no significant difference of yoga on retention for dissimilar pairs of players.

1.i.: There will be no significant difference of yoga on visual retention of players.

1.j.: There will be no significant difference of yoga on recognition of players.

4.2 EFFECTS OF YOGA ON MEMORY OF PLAYERS FROM DIFFERENT UNIVERSITIES

Table 4.2.1: Difference in the results of the PGI memory scale test of the respondents before attending the yoga camp with respect to their universities

ANOVA					
	Sum of Squares	df	Mean Square	F-value	p-value
Between Groups	415.310	3	138.437	3.408	0.021*
Within Groups	3899.440	96	40.619		
Total	4314.750	99			

* 0.05 level of significance

The above table explains the output of one-way ANOVA test which was implemented to investigate the difference in the results of the PGI memory scale test of the players before attending the yoga camp, with respect to their universities. The ANOVA test was used to determine whether there are any statistically significant differences between the means of three or more independent (unrelated) groups. There are players from four different universities of Haryana taken into consideration such as Chaudhary Devi Lal University (CDLU), Sirsa; Chaudhary Ranbir Singh University (CRSU), Jind; Kurukshetra University, Kurukshetra (KUK) and Maharshi Dayanand University (MDU), Rohtak. As shown by the numbers of the above table, with the F-value of 3.408 and p-value of 0.021 (i.e. significant), we can reject the null hypothesis for F-test and can conclude that there was a statistically significant difference in the results of the memory test of the players before attending the yoga camp, belong to different universities of Haryana.

Table 4.2.2: Comparison of the results of the PGI memory scale test of the respondents before attending the yoga camp with respect to their universities

(I) University		Multiple Comparisons				
		Mean Difference (I-J)	Std. Error	p-value	95% Confidence Interval	
					Lower Bound	Upper Bound
CDLU	CRSU	0.200	1.803	0.912	-3.378	3.778
	KUK	-4.880	1.803	0.008**	-8.458	-1.302
	MDU	-1.840	1.803	0.310	-5.418	1.738
CRSU	CDLU	-0.200	1.803	0.912	-3.778	3.378
	KUK	-5.080	1.803	0.006**	-8.658	-1.502
	MDU	-2.040	1.803	0.261	-5.618	1.538
KUK	CDLU	4.880	1.803	0.008**	1.302	8.458
	CRSU	5.080	1.803	0.006**	1.502	8.658
	MDU	3.040	1.803	0.095	-0.538	6.618
MDU	CDLU	1.840	1.803	0.310	-1.738	5.418
	CRSU	2.040	1.803	0.261	-1.538	5.618
	KUK	-3.040	1.803	0.095	-6.618	0.538

*. 0.05 level of significance; **. 0.01 level of significance

The above table compare the results of PGI memory scale test of the players for four different universities such as Chaudhary Devi Lal University (CDLU), Sirsa; Chaudhary Ranbir Singh University (CRSU), Jind; Kurukshetra University, Kurukshetra (KUK) and Maharshi Dayanand University (MDU), Rohtak before attending the yoga camp. We have applied Least Significant Difference (LSD) test to draw the significance of the difference. Granting the above table, KUK and CDLU, and KUK and CRSU, pairs have p-value less than 0.05, hence we can state that the difference of results of memory test of players between these universities was significant. As shown by the mean difference values, players from KUK have higher mean value for memory test as compare to CDLU, and CRSU. On the other hand, the mean difference for rest of the pairs was not significant as the p-value was greater than 0.05.

Table 4.2.3: Difference in the results of the PGI memory scale test of the respondents after attending the yoga camp with respect to their universities

ANOVA					
	Sum of Squares	df	Mean Square	F-value	p-value
Between Groups	375.310	3	125.103	6.169	0.001**
Within Groups	1946.880	96	20.280		
Total	2322.190	99			

**. 0.01 level of significance

The above table explains the output of one-way ANOVA test which was applied to assess the difference in the results of the PGI memory scale test of the players after attending the yoga camp, with respect to their universities. As shown by the figures of the above table, the F-value was 6.169 and p-value of 0.001 which was very strong to reject the null hypothesis of F-test, and hence, we can reject the null hypothesis and can conclude that therewas a highly significant difference in the results of the memory test of the players after attending the yoga camp, belong to different universities of Haryana.

Table 4.2.4: Comparison of the results of the PGI memory scale test of the respondents after attending the yoga camp with respect to their universities

Multiple Comparisons						
(I) University		Mean Difference (I-J)	Std. Error	p-value	95% Confidence Interval	
					Lower Bound	Upper Bound
CDLU	CRSU	0.360	1.274	0.778	-2.168	2.888
	KUK	-4.400	1.274	0.001**	-6.928	-1.872
	MDU	-2.480	1.274	0.054	-5.008	0.048
CRSU	CDLU	-0.360	1.274	0.778	-2.888	2.168
	KUK	-4.760	1.274	0.001**	-7.288	-2.232
	MDU	-2.840	1.274	0.028*	-5.368	-0.312
KUK	CDLU	4.400	1.274	0.001**	1.872	6.928
	CRSU	4.760	1.274	0.001**	2.232	7.288
	MDU	1.920	1.274	0.135	-0.608	4.448
MDU	CDLU	2.480	1.274	0.054	-0.048	5.008
	CRSU	2.840	1.274	0.028*	0.312	5.368
	KUK	-1.920	1.274	0.135	-4.448	0.608

*. 0.05 level of significance; **. 0.01 level of significance

The above table represents the comparison of the results of PGI memory scale test of the players from four different universities such as Chaudhary Devi Lal University (CDLU), Sirsa; Chaudhary Ranbir Singh University (CRSU), Jind; Kurukshetra University, Kurukshetra (KUK) and Maharshi Dayanand University (MDU), Rohtak after attending the yoga camp. We have implemented Least Significant Difference (LSD) test to draw the conclusions. As shown in the above table, KUK and CDLU, KUK and CRSU, and CRSU and MDU pairs have p-value less than 0.05, hence we can conclude that the difference of results of PGI memory scale test of players between these universities was significant. As shown by the mean difference values, players from KUK have higher mean value for memory test as compare to CDLU, and CRSU, whereas players from MDU have higher mean value for memory test as compare to CRSU. On the other hand, the mean difference for rest of the pairs was not significant as the p-value was greater than 0.05. Figure 4.2.1 exhibits the bar graph for mean values of the results of PGI memory scale test before and after attending yoga camp, with respect to the universities.

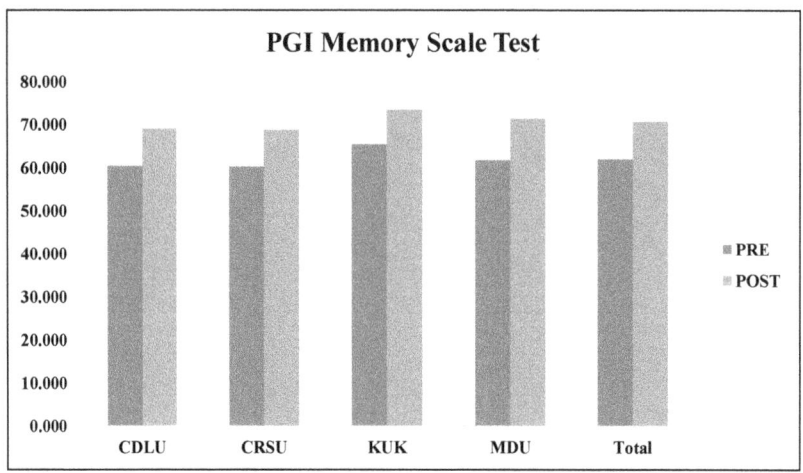

Figure 4.2.1: University wise difference in the mean values of the results of PGI memory scale test for per and posy yoga camp

Table 4.2.5: Difference in the gain in results of the PGI memory scale test of the respondents after attending the yoga camp with respect to their universities

ANOVA						
University	N	Mean	Std. Deviation	F-value	p-value
CDLU	25	8.640	3.546		
CRSU	25	8.480	5.141		
KUK	25	8.160	3.859	0.237	0.870
MDU	25	9.280	6.295		
Total	100	8.640	4.779		

The above table explains the difference in the gain in memory test results after attending the yoga camp. The result was shown with respect to each university. One-way ANOVA was implemented to assess the significance of the difference. As shown in the above table, players from Chaudhary Devi Lal University (CDLU), Sirsa have shown the mean gain of 8.640 with standard deviation 3.546, players of Chaudhary

Ranbir Singh University (CRSU), Jind have shown the mean gain of 8.480 with standard deviation of 5.141, Kurukshetra University, Kurukshetra (KUK) players have shown the mean gain of 8.160 with standard deviation of 3.859, and players from Maharshi Dayanand University (MDU), Rohtak have shown the mean gain of 9.280 with standard deviation of 6.295, in PGI memory scale test. The F-value of 0.237 and p-value 0.870 (non-significant) affirms that we cannot reject the null hypothesis for F-test and can conclude that there was no significant difference in the gain of the results of the PGI memory scale test of the respondents after attending the yoga camp with respect to their universities. Figure 4.2.2 showed the bar plot the gain in PGI memory scale test of the players with respect to their university.

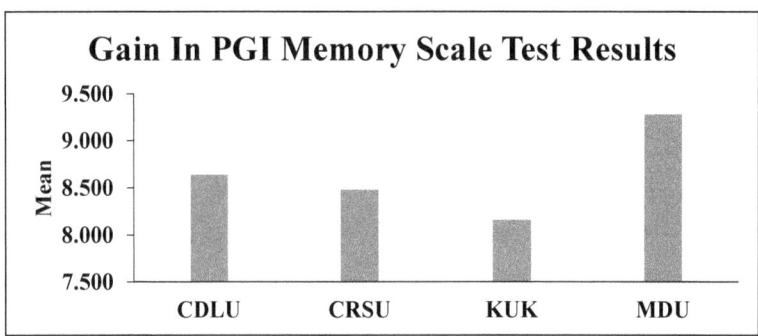

Figure 4.2.2: University wise gain in the PGI memory scale test results

Table 4.2.6: Difference in the results of the PGI memory scale test of the respondents after attending the yoga camp with respect to their universities

		\multicolumn{5}{c}{Paired Samples Statistics}
		N	Mean	Std. Deviation	t-value	p-value
CDLU	PGI PRE	25	60.32	5.68	12.183	0.001**
	PGI POST	25	68.96	4.24		
CRSU	PGI PRE	25	60.12	6.41	8.248	0.001**
	PGI POST	25	68.60	5.06		
KUK	PGI PRE	25	65.20	4.69	10.573	0.001**
	PGI POST	25	73.36	3.93		
PGI	PGI PRE	25	62.16	8.19	7.371	0.001**
	PGI POST	25	71.44	4.71		

**. 0.01 level of significance

The above table exhibits the output of the paired t-test which was applied to investigate the difference in the results of the players from different universities of Haryana for PGI memory scale test, before and after attending the yoga camp. Paired t-test compares the means between two related groups on the same continuous, dependent variable. As shown in the above table, for the players of the Chaudhary Devi Lal University (CDLU), Sirsa t-value was 12.183 with p-value 0.001, which was highly significant, indicate that we can reject the null hypothesis of t-test for CDLU players and can signify that there was a highly significant difference in the performance of PGI memory scale test of players before and after attending the yoga camp. Similarly, for Chaudhary Ranbir Singh University (CRSU), Jind players, the t-value was 8.248 with p-value 0.001 which was very strong to reject the null hypothesis, hence we can state that there was a highly significant difference in the performance of PGI memory scale test of CRSU players before and after attending the yoga camp. The t-value of 10.573 and p-value of 0.001 signify that there was a highly significant difference in the performance of the Kurukshetra University, Kurukshetra (KUK) players in PGI memory scale test, before and after attending the yoga camp. Likewise, for the players Maharshi Dayanand University (MDU), Rohtak t-value was 7.371 with p-value 0.001, since the p-value was less than 0.05, hence we can reject the null hypothesis for MDU players and can infer that there was a highly significant difference in the result of the PGI memory scale test of the MDU players before and after attending the yoga camp.

Since, the p-value of all the variables are highly significant, i.e. less than 0.01, hence we can reject the hypothesis H_1 and can conclude that there was a highly significant difference of yoga on memory of players.

Table 4.2.7: Difference in the results of the remote memory test of the respondents after attending the yoga camp

		N	Mean	Std. Deviation	t-value	p-value
Remote Memory	Pre	100	6.115	1.109	3.124	0.002**
	Post	100	6.462	0.823		

**. 0.01 level of significance

The above table depicts the output of the paired t-test which was implemented to test the difference in the results of the ten subtests such as, remote memory, recent memory, mental balance, attention and concentration, delayed recall, immediate recall, retention for similar pairs, retention for dissimilar pairs, visual retention, and recognition, comes under the PGI memory test scale, before and after attending the yoga camp. Granting the above table, for remote memory test, the t-value was 3.124 with p-value 0.002 which was highly strong to reject the null hypothesis of t-test and can conclude that there was highly significant difference in results of remote memory test of the players, before and after attending the yoga camp. Since, the p-value is less than 0.05, hence we can reject the Ha hypothesis and can conclude that there was a significant difference of yoga on remote memory of players. Figure 4.2.3 exhibits the mean of the results of remote memory test of the players, before and after attending the yoga camp.

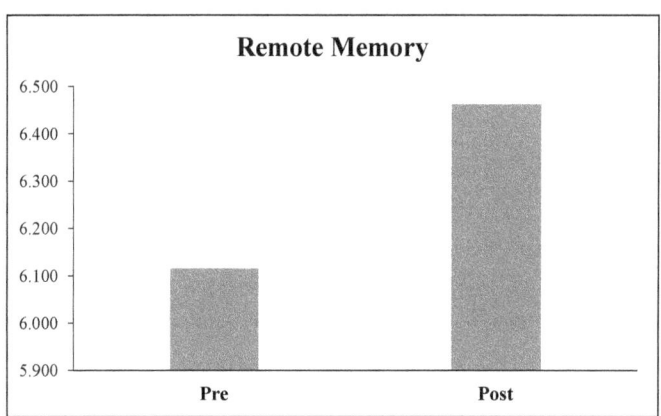

Figure 4.2.3: Mean-wise difference in the performance of the remote memory test of the players, pre and post of attending yoga camp

Table 4.2.8: Difference in the results of the recent memory test of the respondents after attending the yoga camp

		N	Mean	Std. Deviation	t-value	p-value
Recent Memory	Pre	100	5.721	1.136	6.102	0.001**
	Post	100	6.423	0.797		

**. 0.01 level of significance

The t-value for recent memory test was 6.102 with p-value 0.001 (highly significant), hence we can reject the null hypothesis for t-test and can infer that there was highly significant difference in results of recent memory test of the players, before and after attending the yoga camp. Since, the p-value is less than 0.05, hence we can reject the Hb hypothesis and can conclude that there was a significant difference of yoga on recent memory of players. Figure 4.2.4 shows the mean of the results of remote memory test of the players, before and after attending the yoga camp.

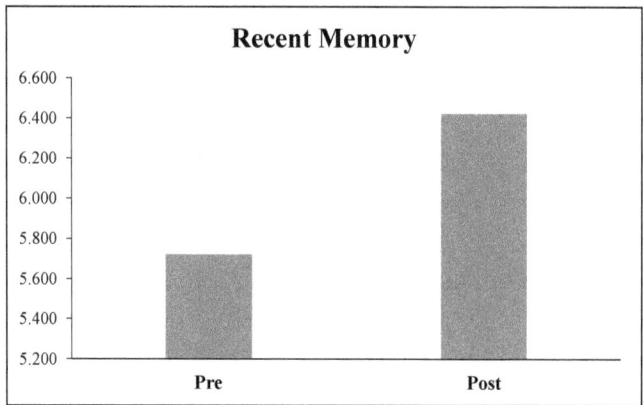

Figure 4.2.4: Mean-wise difference in the performance of the recent memory test of the players, pre and post of attending yoga camp

Table 4.2.9: Difference in the results of the mental balance test of the respondents after attending the yoga camp

		N	Mean	Std. Deviation	t-value	p-value
Mental Balance	Pre	100	7.49	1.468	0.114	0.91
	Post	100	7.51	1.494		

With the t-value of 0.114 and p-value 0.910 for mental balance test, we cannot reject the null hypothesis, hence we accept the null hypothesis of t-test for mental balance, that was, there was no significant difference in the mental balance test of the players for before and after attending the yoga camp. Since, the p-value is greater than 0.05, hence we can accept the Hc hypothesis and can conclude that there was a non-significant difference of yoga on mental balance of players. Figure 4.2.5 explains the mean of the results of mental balance test of the players, before and after attending the yoga camp.

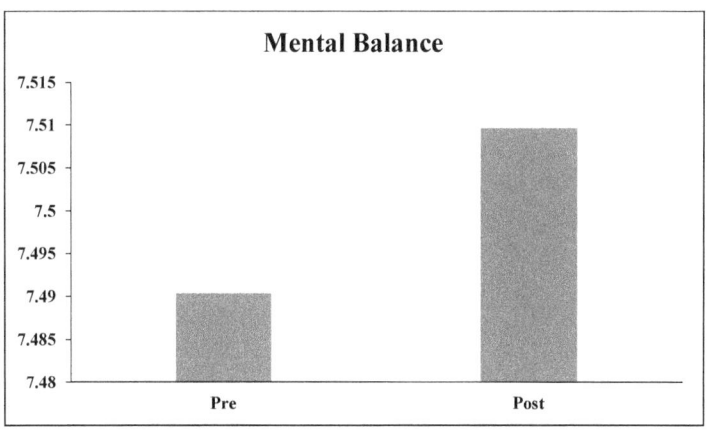

Figure 4.2.5: Mean-wise difference in the performance of the mental balance test of the players, pre and post of attending yoga camp

Table 4.2.10: Difference in the results of the attention and concentration test of the respondents after attending the yoga camp

		N	Mean	Std. Deviation	t-value	p-value
Attention and Concentration	Pre	100	5.375	2.186	1.481	0.142
	Post	100	5.019	1.207		

Similarly, for attention and concentration test, t-value was 1.481 and p-value was 0.142 which was very weak to reject the null hypothesis, hence we can conclude that there was no significant difference in the attention and concentration test of the players, before and after attending the yoga camp. Since, the p-value is greater than 0.05, hence we can accept the Hd hypothesis and can conclude that there was a non-significant difference of yoga on attention and concentration of players. Figure 4.2.6 explains the mean of the results of attention and concentration test of the players, before and after attending the yoga camp.

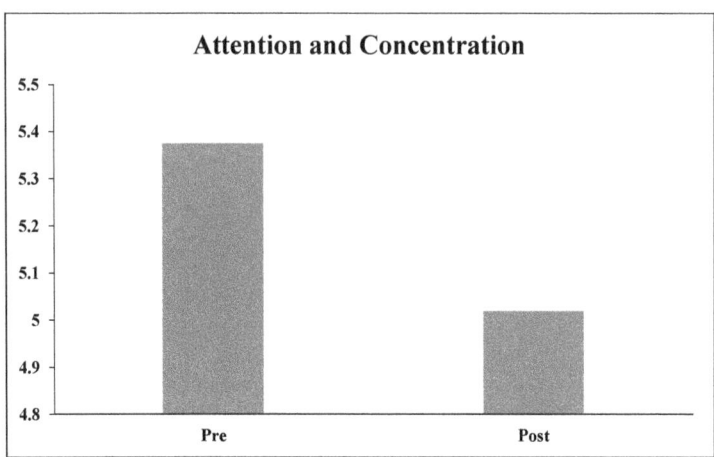

Figure 4.2.6: Mean-wise difference in the performance of the attention and concentration test of the players, pre and post of attending yoga camp

Table 4.2.11: Difference in the results of the delayed recall test of the respondents after attending the yoga camp

		N	Mean	Std. Deviation	t-value	p-value
Delayed Recall	Pre	100	8.538	2.348	5.173	0.001**
	Post	100	9.894	1.386		

**. 0.01 level of significance

On the other hand, for delayed recall test, the t-value was 5.173 with p-value of 0.001 which was highly significant, hence we can reject the null hypothesis of t-test and can conclude that there was a highly significant difference in the results of the delayed recall test of the players for before and after attending the yoga camp. Since, the p-value is less than 0.05, hence we can reject the He, hypothesis and can conclude that there was a significant difference of yoga on delayed recall of players. Figure 4.2.7 shows the mean of the results of delayed recall test of the players, before and after attending the yoga camp.

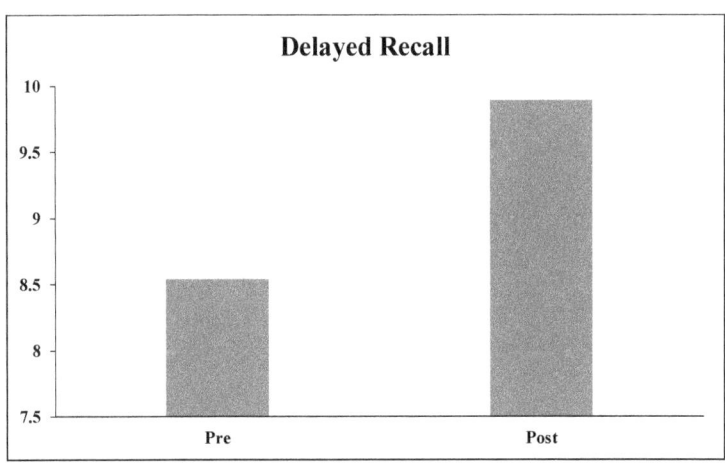

Figure 4.2.7: Mean-wise difference in the performance of the delayed recall test of the players, pre and post of attending yoga camp

Table 4.2.12: Difference in the results of the immediate recall test of the respondents after attending the yoga camp

		N	Mean	Std. Deviation	t-value	p-value
Immediate Recall	Pre	100	8.24	2.977	4.814	0.001**
	Post	100	9.923	2.376		

**. 0.01 level of significance

For immediate recall test, the t-value was 4.814 and p-value was 0.001 which was very strong to reject the null hypothesis of t-test and hence, we can conclude that there was a highly significant difference in the results of the immediate recall test of the players after attending the yoga camp. Since, the p-value is less than 0.05, hence we can reject the Hf hypothesis and can conclude that there was a significant difference of yoga on immediate recall of players. Figure 4.2.8 shows the mean of the results of immediate recall test of the players, before and after attending the yoga camp.

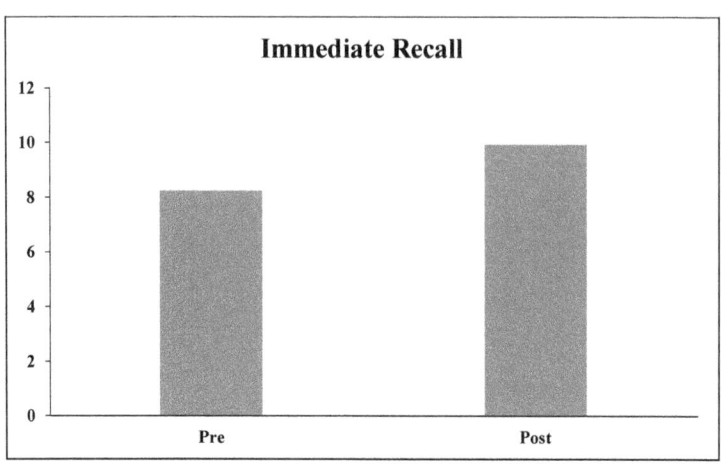

Figure 4.2.8: Mean-wise difference in the performance of the immediate recall test of the players, pre and post of attending yoga camp

Table 4.2.13: Difference in the results of the retention for similar pairs test of the respondents after attending the yoga camp

		N	Mean	Std. Deviation	t-value	p-value
Retention for Similar Pairs	Pre	100	5.837	1.359	0.564	0.574
	Post	100	5.76	0.94		

For retention for similar pairs test, t-value was 0.564 with p-value of 0.574 which was very weak to reject the null hypothesis of t-test, hence we accept the null hypothesis, that was, there was no significant difference in the results of retention for similar pairs test of the players in case of before and after attending the yoga camp. Since, the p-value is greater than 0.05, hence we can accept the Hg hypothesis and can conclude that there was a non-significant difference of yoga on retention for the similar pairs of players. Figure 4.2.9 shows the mean of the results of retention for similar pairs test of the players, before and after attending the yoga camp.

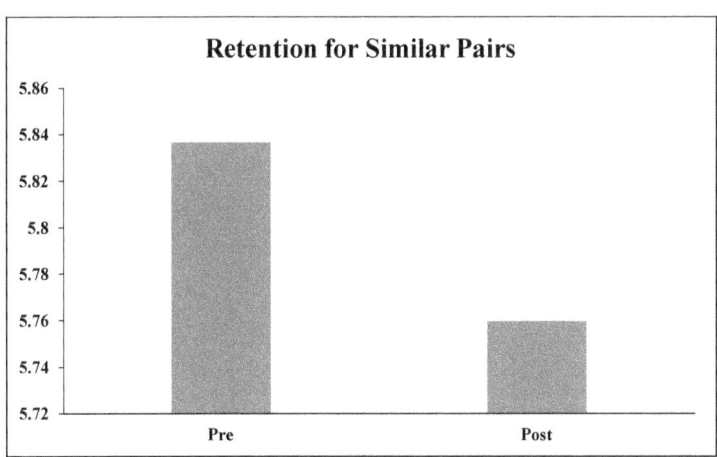

Figure 4.2.9: Mean-wise difference in the performance of the retention for similar pairs test of the players, pre and post of attending yoga camp

Table 4.2.14: Difference in the results of the retention for dissimilar pairs test of the respondents after attending the yoga camp

		N	Mean	Std. Deviation	t-value	p-value
Retention for Dissimilar Pairs	Pre	100	5.019	1.4	18.482	0.001**
	Post	100	10.01	2.354		

**. 0.01 level of significance

For retention for dissimilar pairs test, t-value was 18.482 with p-value of 0.001 which was very strong to reject the null hypothesis of t-test, hence we reject the null hypothesis, that was, there was highly significant difference in the results of retention for dissimilar pairs test of the players, in case of before and after attending the yoga camp. Since, the p-value is less than 0.05, hence we can reject the Hh hypothesis and can conclude that there was a significant difference of yoga on retention for dissimilar pairs of players. Figure 4.2.10 shows the mean of the results of retention for dissimilar pairs test of the players, before and after attending the yoga camp.

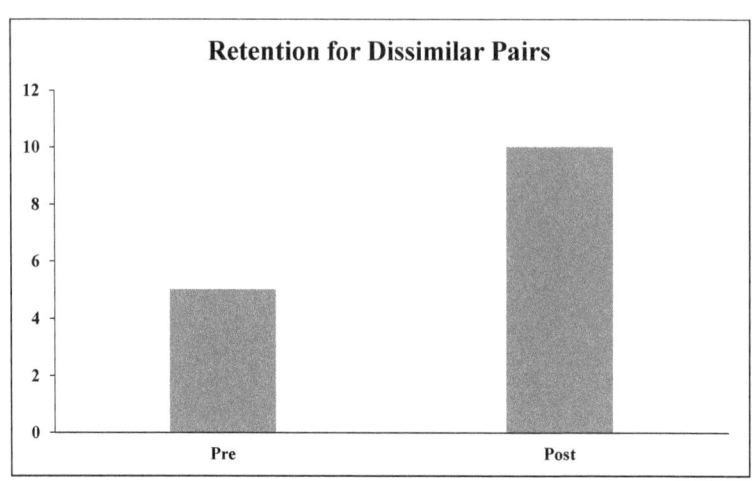

Figure 4.2.10: Mean-wise difference in the performance of the retention for dissimilar pairs test of the players, pre and post of attending yoga camp

Table 4.2.15: Difference in the results of the retention for dissimilar pairs test of the respondents after attending the yoga camp

		N	Mean	Std. Deviation	t-value	p-value
Visual Retention	Pre	100	4.962	1.448	2.091	0.039*
	Post	100	5.26	0.985		

*. 0.05 level of significance

The t-value of 2.091 with p-value 0.039 for visual retention test indicates the significant p-value, hence we can reject the null hypothesis for t-test and can conclude that there was a significant difference in the visual retention test of the players. Since, the p-value is less than 0.05, hence we can reject the Hi, hypothesis and can conclude that there was a significant difference of yoga on visual retention of players. Figure 4.2.11 exhibits the mean of the results of visual retention test of the players, before and after attending the yoga camp.

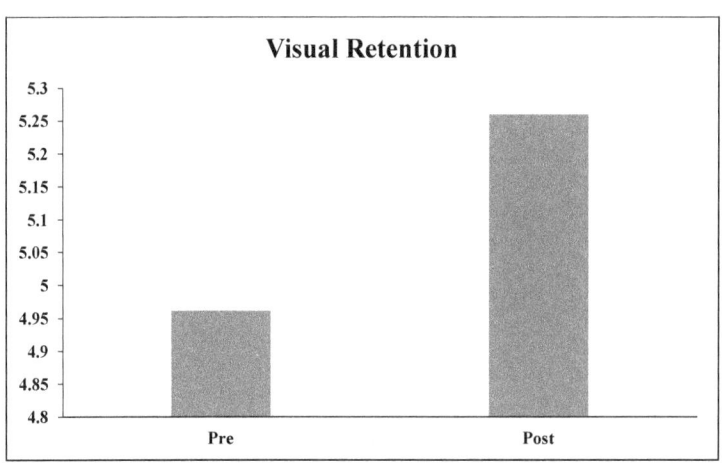

Figure 4.2.11: Mean-wise difference in the performance of the visual retention test of the players, pre and post of attending yoga camp

Table 4.2.16: Difference in the results of the recognition test of the respondents after attending the yoga camp

		N	Mean	Std. Deviation	t-value	p-value
Recognition	Pre	100	4.625	1.345	1.288	0.201
	Post	100	4.442	1.032		

And, for recognition test, with t-value 1.288 and p-value 0.201 we cannot reject the null hypothesis, hence we accept the null hypothesis that there was a non-significant difference in the recognition test of the players for before and after attending the yoga camp. Since, the p-value is greater than 0.05, hence we can accept the Hj, hypothesis and can conclude that there was no significant difference of yoga on recognition capability of the players. Figure 4.2.12 exhibits the mean of the results of recognition test of the players, before and after attending the yoga camp.

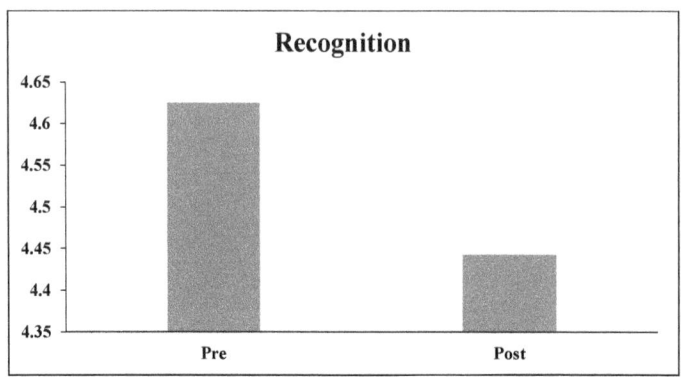

Figure 4.2.12: Mean-wise difference in the performance of the recognition test of the players, pre and post of attending yoga camp

Since, the p-value for variables remote memory, recent memory, delayed recall, immediate recall, retention for dissimilar pairs, and visual retention, was less than 0.05, hence we can reject the Ha, Hb, He, Hf, Hh and Hi, hypotheses and can conclude that there was a significant difference of yoga on remote memory, recent memory, delayed recall, immediate recall, retention for dissimilar pairs, and visual retention of players. On the other hand, the p-value for variables balance, attention and concentration, retention for similar pairs, and recognition, was greater than 0.05, hence we accept the hypotheses Hc, Hd, Hg and Hi, that was, there was a non-significant difference of yoga on balance, attention and concentration, retention for similar pairs, and recognition of players. Figure 4.2.13 showed the bar plot of mean values for ten subtests of PGI memory scale test for pre and post of yoga camp.

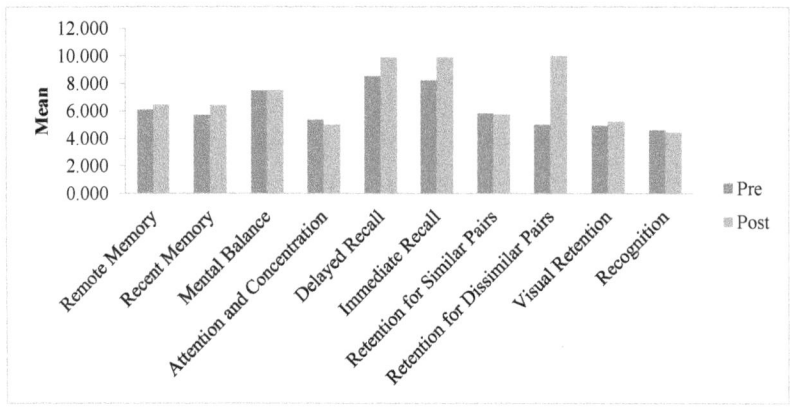

Figure 4.2.13: Difference in the results of ten subtests of PGI memory scale test

OBJECTIVE 2

EFFECTS OF YOGA ON PROBLEM SOLVING ABILITY OF PLAYERS

Hypothesis involved:

H_2: There will be no significant difference of yoga on problem solving ability of players.

4.3 EFFECTS OF YOGASANAS ON PROBLEM SOLVING ABILITY OF PLAYERS

Table 4.3.1: Difference in the results of the problem-solving ability test of the respondents before attending the yoga camp with respect to their universities

	ANOVA				
	Sum of Squares	df	Mean Square	F-value	p-value
Between Groups	68.750	3	22.917	3.142	0.029*
Within Groups	700.240	96	7.294		
Total	768.990	99			

*. 0.05 level of significance

The above table explains the results of the one-way ANOVA test which was implemented to investigate the difference in the results of the problem-solving ability test of the players before attending the yoga camp, with respect to their universities. There are players from four different universities of Haryana taken into consideration such as Chaudhary Devi Lal University (CDLU), Sirsa; Chaudhary Ranbir Singh University (CRSU), Jind; Kurukshetra University, Kurukshetra (KUK) and Maharshi Dayanand University (MDU), Rohtak. As shown by the numbers of the above table, with the F-value of 3.142 and p-value of 0.029 (i.e. significant), we can reject the null hypothesis for F-test and can conclude that there was a statistically significant difference in the results of the problem-solving ability test of the players before attending the yoga camp, belong to different universities of Haryana.

Table 4.3.2: Comparison of the results of the problem-solving ability test of the respondents before attending the yoga camp with respect to their universities

Multiple Comparisons						
UNIVERSITY		Mean Difference (I-J)	Std. Error	p-value	95% Confidence Interval	
					Lower Bound	Upper Bound
CDLU	CRSU	-2.320	0.764	0.003**	-3.836	-0.804
	KUK	-0.880	0.764	0.252	-2.396	0.636
	MDU	-1.160	0.764	0.132	-2.676	0.356
CRSU	CDLU	2.320	0.764	0.003**	0.804	3.836
	KUK	1.440	0.764	0.062	-0.076	2.956
	MDU	1.160	0.764	0.132	-0.356	2.676
KUK	CDLU	0.880	0.764	0.252	-0.636	2.396
	CRSU	-1.440	0.764	0.062	-2.956	0.076
	MDU	-0.280	0.764	0.715	-1.796	1.236
MDU	CDLU	1.160	0.764	0.132	-0.356	2.676
	CRSU	-1.160	0.764	0.132	-2.676	0.356
	KUK	0.280	0.764	0.715	-1.236	1.796

**. 0.01 level of significance

The above table represents the comparison the results of problem-solving ability test of the players from four different universities such as Chaudhary Devi Lal University (CDLU), Sirsa; Chaudhary Ranbir Singh University (CRSU), Jind; Kurukshetra University, Kurukshetra (KUK) and Maharshi Dayanand University (MDU), Rohtak before attending the yoga camp. We have applied Least Significant Difference (LSD) test to draw the significance of the difference. Granting the above table, only CRSU and CDLU pair has p-value less than 0.05 i.e. 0.003, hence we can state that the difference of results of problem-solving ability test of players between these universities was significant. As shown by the mean difference values, players from CRSU has higher mean value for problem-solving ability test as compare to CDLU. On the other hand, the mean difference for rest of the pairs was not significant as the p-value was greater than 0.05.

Table 4.3.3: Difference in the results of the problem-solving ability test of the respondents after attending the yoga camp with respect to their universities

ANOVA					
	Sum of Squares	df	Mean Square	F-value	p-value
Between Groups	96.560	3.000	32.187	6.301	0.001**
Within Groups	490.400	96.000	5.108		
Total	586.960	99.000			

**. 0.01 level of significance

The above table explains the output of one-way ANOVA test which was implemented to investigate the difference in the results of the problem-solving ability test of the players after attending the yoga camp, with respect to their universities. As shown by the figures of the above table, the F-value was 6.301 and p-value of 0.001 which was very strong to reject the null hypothesis of F-test, and hence, we can reject the null hypothesis and can conclude that there was a highly significant difference in the results of the problem-solving ability of the players after attending the yoga camp, belong to different universities of Haryana.

Table 4.3.4: Comparison of the results of the problem-solving ability test of the respondents after attending the yoga camp with respect to their universities

Multiple Comparisons						
UNIVERSITY		Mean Difference (I-J)	Std. Error	p-value	95% Confidence Interval	
					Lower Bound	Upper Bound
CDLU	CRSU	-1.880	0.639	0.004**	-3.149	-0.611
	KUK	-2.600	0.639	0.001**	-3.869	-1.331
	MDU	-2.080	0.639	0.002**	-3.349	-0.811
CRSU	CDLU	1.880	0.639	0.004**	0.611	3.149
	KUK	-0.720	0.639	0.263	-1.989	0.549
	MDU	-0.200	0.639	0.755	-1.469	1.069
KUK	CDLU	2.600	0.639	0.001**	1.331	3.869
	CRSU	0.720	0.639	0.263	-0.549	1.989
	MDU	0.520	0.639	0.418	-0.749	1.789
MDU	CDLU	2.080	0.639	0.002**	0.811	3.349
	CRSU	0.200	0.639	0.755	-1.069	1.469
	KUK	-0.520	0.639	0.418	-1.789	0.749

**. 0.01 level of significance

The above table represents the comparison of the results of problem-solving ability test of the players from four different universities such as Chaudhary Devi Lal University (CDLU), Sirsa; Chaudhary Ranbir Singh University (CRSU), Jind; Kurukshetra University, Kurukshetra (KUK) and Maharshi Dayanand University (MDU), Rohtak after attending the yoga camp. We have implemented Least Significant Difference (LSD) test to draw the conclusions. As shown in the above table, CDLU and CRSU, CDLU and KUK, and CDLU and MDU, pairs have p-value less than 0.05, hence we can conclude that the difference of results of problem-solving ability test of players between these universities was significant. As shown by the mean difference values, players from CDLU have lower mean value for problem-solving ability test as compare to CRSU, KUK and MDU. On the other hand, the mean difference for rest of the pairs was not significant as the p-value was greater than 0.05. Figure 4.3.1 exhibits the bar graph for mean values of the results of problem-solving ability test before and after attending yoga camp, with respect to the universities.

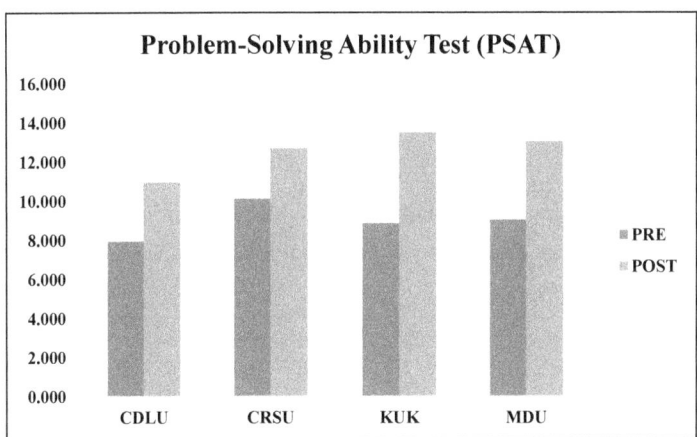

Figure 4.3.1: University wise difference in the mean values of the results of problem-solving ability test for per and posy yoga camp

Table 4.3.5: Difference in the gain in results of the problem-solving ability test of the respondents after attending the yoga camp with respect to their universities

ANOVA					
University	N	Mean	Std. Deviation	F-value	p-value
CDLU	25	2.960	1.369	4.346	0.006**
CRSU	25	2.520	2.417		
KUK	25	4.680	3.224		
MDU	25	3.880	1.810		
Total	100	3.510	2.427		

**. 0.01 level of significance

The above table explains the difference in the gain in problem-solving ability results after attending the yoga camp. The result was shown with respect to each university. One-way ANOVA was implemented to assess the significance of the difference. As shown in the above table, players from CDLU have shown the mean gain of 2.960 with standard deviation 1.369, players of CRSU have shown the mean gain of 2.520 with standard deviation of 2.417, KUK players have shown the mean gain of 4.680 with standard deviation of 3.224, and players from MDU have shown the mean gain of 3.880 with standard deviation of 1.810, in problem-solving ability test. The F-value of 4.304 and p-value 0.007 (highly significant) indicates that we can reject the null hypothesis for F-test and can conclude that there was a highly significant difference in the gain of the results of the problem-solving ability test of the respondents after attending the yoga camp with respect to their universities.

Table 4.3.6: Comparison of the gain in the results of the problem-solving ability test of the respondents after attending the yoga camp with respect to their universities

Multiple Comparisons						
UNIVERSITY		Mean Difference (I-J)	Std. Error	p-value	95% Confidence Interval	
					Lower Bound	Upper Bound
CDLU	CRSU	0.440	0.654	0.503	-0.858	1.738
	KUK	-1.720	0.654	0.010**	-3.018	-0.422
	MDU	-0.920	0.654	0.163	-2.218	0.378
CRSU	CDLU	-0.440	0.654	0.503	-1.738	0.858
	KUK	-2.160	0.654	0.001**	-3.458	-0.862
	MDU	-1.360	0.654	0.040*	-2.658	-0.062
KUK	CDLU	1.720	0.654	0.010**	0.422	3.018
	CRSU	2.160	0.654	0.001**	0.862	3.458
	MDU	0.800	0.654	0.224	-0.498	2.098
MDU	CDLU	0.920	0.654	0.163	-0.378	2.218
	CRSU	1.360	0.654	0.040*	0.062	2.658
	KUK	-0.800	0.654	0.224	-2.098	0.498

*. 0.05 level of significance; **. 0.01 level of significance

The above table compares the gain in the results of problem-solving ability test of the players from four different universities such as Chaudhary Devi Lal University (CDLU), Sirsa; Chaudhary Ranbir Singh University (CRSU), Jind; Kurukshetra University, Kurukshetra (KUK) and Maharshi Dayanand University (MDU), Rohtak after attending the yoga camp. We have implemented Least Significant Difference (LSD) test to draw the significance of difference. As shown in the above table, CDLU and KUK, CRSU and KUK, and CRSU and MDU, pairs have p-value less than 0.05, hence we can conclude that the difference of the gain in the results of problem-solving ability test of players between these universities was significant. As shown by the mean difference values, players from KUK have higher mean value for gain in problem-solving ability test as compare to CRSU, and CDLU, whereas players from MDU have higher mean value as compare to CRSU. On the other hand, the mean difference for rest of the pairs was not significant as the p-value was greater than 0.05. Figure 4.3.2 shows the bar plot the gain in problem-solving ability test of the players with respect to their university.

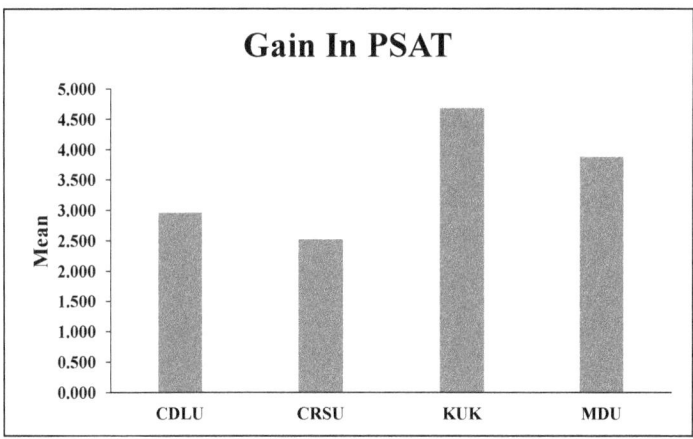

Figure 4.3.2: University wise gain in the problem-solving ability test results

Table 4.3.7: Difference in the results of the problem-solving ability test of the players after attending the yoga camp with respect to their universities

		\multicolumn{5}{c}{Paired Samples Statistics}			
		N	Mean	Std. Deviation	t-value	p-value
CDLU	PSAT PRE	25	7.92	1.98	10.813	0.001**
	PSAT POST	25	10.88	2.01		
CRSU	PSAT PRE	25	10.24	3.42	5.212	0.001**
	PSAT POST	25	12.76	2.45		
KUK	PSAT PRE	25	8.80	2.66	7.258	0.001**
	PSAT POST	25	13.48	2.60		
PGI	PSAT PRE	25	9.08	2.55	10.717	0.001**
	PSAT POST	25	12.96	1.90		

**. 0.01 level of significance

The above table showed the output of the paired t-test which was applied to see whether the difference in the results of the players from different universities of Haryana for problem-solving ability test, before and after attending the yoga camp was significant or not. Paired t-test compares the means between two related groups on the same continuous, dependent variable. As shown in the above table, for the players of the Chaudhary Devi Lal University (CDLU), Sirsa t-value was 10.813 with p-value 0.001, which was highly significant, indicate that we can reject the null hypothesis of t-test for CDLU players and can signify that there was a highly significant difference in the performance of problem-solving ability test of players, before and after attending the yoga camp. Similarly, for Chaudhary Ranbir Singh University (CRSU), Jind players, the t-value was 5.212 with p-value 0.001 which was very strong to reject the null hypothesis, hence we can state that there was a highly significant difference in the performance of problem-solving ability test of CRSU players before and after attending the yoga camp. The t-value of 7.258 and p-value of 0.001 signify that there was a highly significant difference in the performance of the Kurukshetra University, Kurukshetra (KUK) players in problem-solving ability test, before and after attending the yoga camp. Likewise, for the players Maharshi Dayanand University (MDU), Rohtak t-value was 10.717 with p-value 0.001, since the p-value was less than 0.05, hence we can reject the null hypothesis for MDU players and can infer that there was a highly significant difference in the result of the problem-solving ability test of the MDU players before and after attending the yoga camp.

Since, the p-value of all the variables are highly significant, i.e. less than 0.01, hence we can reject the hypothesis H_2 and can conclude that there was a highly significant difference of yoga on problem-solving ability of players.

OBJECTIVE 3

CORRELATION BETWEEN MEMORY AND PROBLEM-SOLVING ABILITY OF PLAYERS

Hypothesis involved:

H_3: There will be no significant correlation between memory and problem-solving ability of players.

4.4 CORRELATION BETWEEN MEMORY AND PROBLEM-SOLVING ABILITY

Table 4.4.1: Correlation between results of the PGI memory scale test and problem-solving ability test of players from different universities of Haryana before attending the yoga camp

Correlations				
UNIVERSITY			PGI PRE	PSAT PRE
CDLU	PGI PRE	Pearson Correlation	1.000	0.014
		p-value		0.946
	PSAT PRE	Pearson Correlation	0.014	1.000
		p-value	0.946	
CRSU	PGI PRE	Pearson Correlation	1.000	0.233
		p-value		0.252
	PSAT PRE	Pearson Correlation	0.233	1.000
		p-value	0.252	
KUK	PGI PRE	Pearson Correlation	1.000	0.333
		p-value		0.097
	PSAT PRE	Pearson Correlation	0.333	1.000
		p-value	0.097	
MDU	PGI PRE	Pearson Correlation	1.000	0.096
		p-value		0.639
	PSAT PRE	Pearson Correlation	0.096	1.000
		p-value	0.639	

The above table depicts the Pearson correlation between the memory and problem-solving ability of players from four different universities such as Chaudhary Devi Lal University (CDLU), Sirsa; Chaudhary Ranbir Singh University (CRSU), Jind; Kurukshetra University, Kurukshetra (KUK) and Maharshi Dayanand University (MDU), Rohtak before attending the yoga camp. The Pearson's correlation coefficientis a measure of the strength and direction of association that exists between two variables. The value lies between +1 and -1, where +1 refers to higher positive correlation, -1 signifies the higher negative correlation and 0 stands for no correlation. As shown by the above table, for CDLU, there was a non-significant (p-value > 0.05) positive correlation between result of the memory and problem-solving ability test of the players, with correlation efficient of 0.014. Similarly, result of PGI memory scale test of players was positively correlated with results of the problem-solving ability test with correlation coefficient of 0.233, but the correlation was non-significant as the p-values was greater than 0.05. For KUK, there was a non-significant (p-value > 0.05) positive correlation between result of the memory and problem-solving ability test of the players, with correlation efficient of 0.333. Likewise, result of PGI memory scale test of players was positively correlated with results of the problem-solving ability test with correlation coefficient of 0.096, but the correlation was non-significant as the p-values was greater than 0.05.

Table 4.4.2: Correlation between results of the PGI memory scale test and problem-solving ability test of players from different universities of Haryana after attending the yoga camp

Correlations				
UNIVERSITY			PGI POST	PSAT POST
CDLU	PGI POST	Pearson Correlation	1.000	0.010
		p-value		0.962
	PSAT POST	Pearson Correlation	0.010	1.000
		p-value	0.962	
CRSU	PGI POST	Pearson Correlation	1.000	0.339
		p-value		0.090
		N	26.000	26.000
	PSAT POST	Pearson Correlation	0.339	1.000
		p-value	0.090	
KUK	PGI POST	Pearson Correlation	1.000	0.385
		p-value		0.052
	PSAT POST	Pearson Correlation	0.385	1.000
		p-value	0.052	
MDU	PGI POST	Pearson Correlation	1.000	0.134
		p-value		0.513
	PSAT POST	Pearson Correlation	0.134	1.000
		p-value	0.513	

The above table depicts the Pearson correlation between the memory and problem-solving ability of players from four different universities such as Chaudhary Devi Lal University (CDLU), Sirsa; Chaudhary Ranbir Singh University (CRSU), Jind; Kurukshetra University, Kurukshetra (KUK) and Maharshi Dayanand University (MDU), Rohtak after attending the yoga camp. As shown by the figures of the above table, for CDLU, there was a non-significant (p-value > 0.05) positive correlation between result of the memory and problem-solving ability test of the players, with correlation efficient of 0.010. Similarly, result of PGI memory scale test of players was positively correlated with results of the problem-solving ability test with correlation coefficient of 0.339, but the correlation was non-significant as the p-values was greater than 0.05. For KUK, there was a non-significant (p-value > 0.05) positive correlation between result of the memory and problem-solving ability test of the players, with correlation efficient of 0.385. Likewise, result of PGI memory scale test of players was positively correlated with results of the problem-solving ability test with correlation coefficient of 0.134, but the correlation was non-significant as the p-values was greater than 0.05.

Since, the p-value for the results of PGI memory scale test and problem-solving ability test of players from four different universities of Haryana, was coming out to be greater than 0.05 for both, before and after attending the yoga camp, hence we cannot reject the H_3 hypothesis. Therefore, we accept the H_3 hypothesis that was, there was no significant correlation between the memory and problem-solving ability of players.

CHAPTER 5

RESULT, CONCLUSION AND RECOMMENDATIONS

The process of analysing and interpreting data, this study would be incomplete if it did not include recommendations. This chapter contains the conclusions as well as the evidence that supports them. It is based on information. On what are the various findings based. The range of application of the conclusions is also specified based on the sample, technique, and collecting and analysis of data restrictions. Conclusions do not solely consist of positive outcomes; no outcomes are also well-represented in this chapter. Following that, this chapter includes recommendations for additional research. All of the findings that developed during the research process are referred to as research recommendations. Along with providing answers to certain difficulties, the research also raises new questions that might be utilized to suggest for further studies.

5.1 DISCUSSION OF THE RESULTS

On the basis of the statistical analyses of the data, the results were as follows.

There will be no significant difference of yoga on memory of players after study we had rejected the null hypothesis for F-test and can presume that there was a measurably huge distinction in the after effects of the memory trial of the players prior to going to the yoga camp, had a place with various universities of Haryana. A few investigations had featured the mental, for instance, Schaeffer (2002) guaranteed "yoga can forestall memory slips by quieting you and improving your fixation. It can likewise improve your forces of review by expanding dissemination to your mind." Specifically, two rearranged presents are recommended, the open-legged forward bend and threading the needle.

There will be no significant difference of yoga on remote memory of players. After analysis of the study for remote memory test, the t-value was 3.124 with p-value 0.002 which was highly strong to reject the null hypothesis of t-test and conclude that there was highly significant difference in results of remote memory test of the players, before and after attending the yoga camp. Result of this study was almost in line with our study, Shashi (1989) used five intellectual tests (shading abrogation, digit forward, digit in reverse, acknowledgment, and visual maintenance) to contemplate the impacts of yoga over the period of time of a scholastic year for 12 year old members. Results showed enhancement for most tests from the start to the furthest limit of the school year both for a gathering that routinely took an interest in yoga and a gathering that did not accepted.

There will be no significant difference of yoga on recent memory of players of players, the t-value for recent memory test was 6.102 with p-value 0.001 (highly significant), hence we could reject the null hypothesis for t-test and can infer that there was highly significant difference in results of recent memory test of the players, before and after attending the yoga camp. The effect of yogic exercise on the mind is aid to have immediate effects. Kocher (1979) used both meaningful words and nonsense syllables to test immediate (short-term) verbal memory abilities before and after a one-month period of yoga training for college-aged males and females. The results, though incomplete, suggested that yoga did facilitate immediate memory performance more than the absence of yoga, and that the benefit was greater for males than for females.

There will be no significant difference of yoga on mental balance of players. With the t-value of 0.114 and p-value 0.910 for mental balance test, we could not reject the null hypothesis, hence we accept the null hypothesis of t-test for mental balance, and there was no significant difference in the mental balance test of the players for before and after attending the yoga camp. Present study also shows that Yoga has become a very popular recreational activity for many Americans. A relationship between the practice of yoga and benefits related to mental balance and overall wellness is apparent (Schaeffer, 2002).

There will be no significant difference of yoga on attention and concentration of players. Similarly, for attention and concentration test, t-value was 1.481 and p-value was 0.142 which was very weak to reject the null hypothesis, hence we conclude that there was no significant difference in the attention and concentration test of the players, before and after attending the yoga camp. Moreover, changes were seen on attention and concentration level of yoga players after three months of yoga training. These findings were almost in line with the result of this study specifically, inverted yogsa position have been associated with claims of increased memory and attention due to increased blood flow to the brain. For example, Schaeffer (2002) claimed "yoga can prevent memory lapses by claiming you and enhancing your concentration. All mentioned studies found similar results on the attention and concentration of players after yoga trainings. The findings of the study were in agreement with the results of Das (2019), Kallivayalil (2021).

There will be no significant difference of yoga on delayed recall of players. The t-value was 5.173 with p-value of 0.001 which was highly significant; hence we could reject the null hypothesis of t-test and conclude that there was a highly significant difference in the results of the delayed recall test of the players for before and after attending the yoga camp. NK, M., & Telles, S. (2004) the purpose of the study was to find out the effect of Spatial and verbal memory test scores following yoga and fine arts camps for school children. The groups of thirty students equally divided into two groups and aged 11 to 16 years were there. One group attended a yoga camp and the other a fine arts camp. Both groups were assessed on the memory tasks pre and after ten days of their respective interventions. A control group (n= 30) was similarly studied to assess the test–retest effect. At the final assessment the yoga group showed a significant increase of 43% in spatial memory scores (Multivariate analysis, Tukey test), while the fine arts and control groups showed no change. The results suggested that yoga practice, including physical postures, yoga breathing, meditation and guided relaxation improved delayed recall of spatial information.

There will be no significant difference of yoga on immediate recall of players. The t-value was 4.814 and p-value is 0.001which was very strong to reject the null hypothesis of t-test and hence, we could conclude that there was a highly significant difference in the results of the immediate recall test of the players after attending the yoga camp. The effect of yogic exercises on the mind is said to have immediate effects. Kocher (1974) used both meaningful words and nonsense syllables to test immediate (short-term) verbal memory abilities before and after a one-month period of yoga training for college-aged males and females. The results, though incomplete, suggested that yoga did facilitate immediate memory performance more than the absence of yoga, and that the benefit was greater for males than for females.

There will be no significant difference of yoga on retention for similar pairs of players. The t-value was 0.564 with p-value of 0.574 which was very weak to reject the null hypothesis of t-test, hence we accept the null hypothesis, so there was no significant difference in the results of retention for similar pairs test of the players in case of before and after attending the yoga camp Sahasi (1989) utilized five cognitive tests (color cancellation, digit forward, digit backward, recognition, and visual retention) to study the effects of yoga over the time span of an academic year for 12 year old participants. Results showed improvement on most tests from the beginning to the end of the school year both for a group that regularly participated in yoga and a group that did not.

There will be no significant difference of yoga on retention for dissimilar pairs of players. The t-value was 18.482 with p-value of 0.001 which was very strong to reject the null hypothesis of t-test, hence we reject the null hypothesis, and so there was highly significant difference in the results of retention for dissimilar pair's test of the players, in case of before and after attending the yoga camp. Kioumourtzoglou et al. (1998) "aim of this study to assess cognitive, perceptual and motor skill ability in elite Basketball players". Thirteen (n-13) men of elite male national team of Basketball players were selected as a sample for laboratory study aged lies between 22 to 23 years and fifteen men of same age (physical education class) were selected to assess difference in their scores on cognitive skill (memory-retention, memory grouping analytics ability), perceptual skill (speed of perception, prediction, selective attention, response selection and motor skills (dynamic balance, whole body coordination, wrist - finger dexterity, rhythmic ability). The result shows that those who are elite Basketball players score better on memory-retention, selective attention, and on prediction measures than the control group.

There will be no significant difference of yoga on visual retention of players. The t-value of 2.091 with p-value 0.039 for visual retention test indicates the significant p-value, hence we could reject the null hypothesis for t-test and conclude that there was a significant difference in the visual retention. It was evident from the above finding that test of the players Cowen and Adams (2005) have evaluated the impact of six weeks of either ashtanga yoga or hatha yoga classes. Significant improvements in follow-up were observed in all participants in diastolic blood pressure, upper body and stem muscle strength and endurance, flexibility, visual stress, and health perception. Progress given by each group compared to basic tests. The group of astanga yoga has lowered diastolic blood pressure and visual acuity, and increased body and stem muscle strength and endurance, flexibility, and a sense of well-being. The development of the hatha yoga group was only important for trunk muscle strength and endurance and flexibility. The findings suggest that the benefits of practicing yoga vary in style.

There will be no significant difference of yoga on recognition of players for recognition test, with t-value 1.288 and p-value 0.201 we could not reject the null hypothesis; hence we accept the null hypothesis that there was a non-significant difference in the recognition test of the players for before and after attending the yoga camp. Raingruber (2007) the outcomes of the self-care classes described by nurses include: (a) awareness of warmth, tingling, and relaxation, (b) awareness of improved problem-solving ability, and (c) recognition of increased ability to focus on patient needs. Hospitals willing to invest in nursing care options can expect patient and work-related benefits. The scientific studies related Kioumourtzoglou et al (1998) aim of this study to assess cognitive, perceptual and motor skill ability in elite Basketball players. Thirteen (n-13) men of elite male national team of Basketball players were selected as a sample for laboratory study aged lies between 22 to 23 years and fifteen men of same age (physical education class) were selected to assess difference in their scores on cognitive skill (memory-retention, memory grouping analytics ability), perceptual skill speed of perception, prediction, selective attention, response selection and motor skills (dynamic balance, whole body coordination, wrist - finger dexterity, rhythmic ability). The result shows that those who are elite Basketball players score better on memory-retention, selective attention, and on prediction measures than the control group. NK, M., & Telles, S. (2004) the purpose of the study was to find out the effect of Spatial and verbal memory test scores following yoga and fine arts camps for school children. The groups of thirty students equally divided into two groups and aged 11 to 16 years were there. One group attended a yoga camp and the other a fine arts camp. Both groups were assessed on the memory tasks pre and after ten days of their respective interventions. A control group (n= 30) was similarly studied to assess the test–retest effect. At the final assessment the yoga group showed a significant increase of 43% in spatial memory scores (Multivariate analysis, Tukey test), while the fine arts and control groups showed no change. The results suggested that yoga practice, including physical postures, yoga breathing, and meditation and guided relaxation improved delayed recall of spatial information.

There will be no significant difference of yoga on problem solving ability of players. We could reject the null hypothesis for F-test and can conclude that there was a statistically significant difference in the results of the problem-solving ability test of the players before attending the yoga camp, belong to different universities of Haryana. Fatin Abdullah et al. (2005) investigated physics problem solving skills of secondary students in relation to ethnicity. Five students achieving the highest scores on both the Physics Problems Solving Ability Test (PPSAT) and the Metacognitive Skills Questionnaire (MSQ) were selected to be reassessed using the qualitative techniques. The qualitative techniques are thinking aloud protocol, interviews and analysis of the paper & pencil test by the students. The cross tabulation and triangulation techniques were implied and the results were later being compared with the past researches found in the literature. This study was conducted in Malaysia. It was found that ethnicity has a significant effect on the problem solving ability of secondary students. It was observed that Chinese students have more magnitude of problem solving skills as compared to Malay students but no significant difference was observed in problem solving skills of Indian and Chinese as well as Indian and Malay students. The results showed a partial effect of ethnicity on problem solving skills of secondary students.

There will be no significant correlation between memory and problem-solving ability of players. Likewise, result of PGI memory scale test of players was positively correlated with results of the problem-solving ability test with correlation coefficient of 0.096, but the correlation was non-significant as the p-values was greater than 0.05. Before and after attending the yoga camp, hence we could not reject the Hypothesis 3. Therefore, we accept the H03 hypothesis, so there was no significant correlation between the memory and problem-solving ability of players. It was evident from the above finding that Shahbazi (2018) studied the effect of problem solving skill training on emotional intelligence of nursing students. Heidari (2016) studied the effect of problem solving training on decision –making skill and critical thinking in emergency medical personnel.

5.2 CONCLUSION

The following conclusion was drawn under the light of the study.

Hypothesis No.1: There will be no significant difference of yoga on memory of players after study we had rejected the null hypothesis for F-test and conclude that there was a statistically significant difference in the results of the memory test of the players before and after attending the yoga camp, belong to different universities of Haryana

Hypothesis 1.a: There will be no significant difference of yoga on remote memory of players. After analysis of study for remote memory test, the t-value was 3.124 with p-value 0.002 which was highly strong to reject the null hypothesis of t-test and conclude that there was highly significant difference in results of remote memory test of the players, before and after attending the yoga camp.

Hypothesis 1.b: There will be no significant difference of yoga on recent memory of players. The t-value for recent memory test was 6.102 with p-value 0.001 (highly significant), hence we can reject the null hypothesis for t-test and can infer that there was highly significant difference in results of recent memory test of the players, before and after attending the yoga camp.

Hypothesis 1.c: There will be no significant difference of yoga on mental balance of players. With the t-value of 0.114 and p-value 0.910 for mental balance test, we could not reject the null hypothesis, hence we accepted the null hypothesis of t-test for mental balance, so there was no significant difference in the mental balance test of the players for before and after attending the yoga camp.

Hypothesis 1.d: There will be no significant difference of yoga on attention and concentration of players. Similarly, for attention and concentration test, t-value was 1.481 and p-value was 0.142 which was very weak to reject the null hypothesis, hence we would conclude that there was no significant difference in the attention and concentration test of the players, before and after attending the yoga camp.

Hypothesis 1.e: There will be no significant difference of yoga on delayed recall of players. On the other hand, for delayed recall test, the t-value was 5.173 with p-value of 0.001 which was highly significant, hence we would reject the null hypothesis of t-test and conclude that there was a highly significant difference in the results of the delayed recall test of the players for before and after attending the yoga camp.

Hypothesis 1.f: There will be no significant difference of yoga on immediate recall of players. For immediate recall test, the t-value was 4.814 and p-value was 0.001which was very strong to reject the null hypothesis of t-test and hence, we would conclude that there was a highly significant difference in the results of the immediate recall test of the players after attending the yoga camp.

Hypothesis 1.g: There will be no significant difference of yoga on retention for similar pairs of players. For retention for similar pairs test, t-value was 0.564 with p-value of 0.574 which was very weak to reject the null hypothesis of t-test, hence we accept the null hypothesis, so there was no significant difference in the results of retention for similar pairs test of the players in case of before and after attending the yoga camp

Hypothesis 1.h: There will be no significant difference of yoga on retention for dissimilar pairs of players. For retention for dissimilar pairs test, t-value was 18.482 with p-value of 0.001 which was very strong to reject the null hypothesis of t-test, hence we reject the null hypothesis, so there was highly significant difference in the results of retention for dissimilar pairs test of the players, in case of before and after attending the yoga camp.

Hypothesis 1.i: There will be no significant difference of yoga on visual retention of players. The t-value of 2.091 with p-value 0.039 for visual retention test indicates the significant p-value; hence we would reject the null hypothesis for t-test and conclude that there was a significant difference in the visual retention test of the players

Hypothesis 1.j: There will be no significant difference of yoga on recognition of players. For recognition test, with t-value 1.288 and p-value 0.201 we could not reject the null hypothesis, hence we accept the null hypothesis that there was a non-significant difference in the recognition test of the players for before and after attending the yoga camp.

Hypothesis 2: There will be no significant difference of yoga on problem solving ability of players. We could reject the null hypothesis for F-test and conclude that there was a statistically significant difference in the results of the problem-solving ability test of the players before attending the yoga camp, belong to different universities of Haryana.

Hypothesis 3: There will be no significant correlation between memory and problem-solving ability of players. Likewise, result of PGI memory scale test of players was positively correlated with results of the problem-solving ability test with correlation coefficient of 0.096, but the correlation was non-significant as the p-values was greater than 0.05. Before and after attending the yoga camp, hence we could not reject the Hypothesis 3. Therefore, we accept the Hypothesis 3 so; there was no significant correlation between the memory and problem-solving ability of players.

5.3 RECOMMENDATION FOR FURTHER STUDIES

The following recommendations were made on the basis of the study:

- The similar study may be conducted by using other types of yogasana training programme.
- The similar study may be carried out by using the larger sample size and other age group.
- The similar study may be carried out by using different duration of training programme.
- The similar study may be conducted for other topographical areas of the state and nation.
- Similar studies may be conducted selecting other sociopsychological and economic groups.

SUMMARY

Yoga is a pragmatic comprehensive way of thinking intended to achieve significant state too is a vital subject, which contemplates man all in all. The point of Yoga is to devise available resources of aiding the better passionate and scholarly focus. Yoga deals with all parts of the individual: the physical, mental, enthusiastic, mystic and profound. Today, yoga being a subject of shifted interests, has acquired overall ubiquity. Late examination patterns have shown that it can fill in as an applied science in various fields like training, actual schooling and sports, wellbeing and family government assistance, brain research and medication and furthermore one of the methods for the presentation and usefulness. Investigates in the field of yoga have set up that the yogic asana, pranayamas and kriyas are the awesome valuable as they help not exclusively to reinforce every organ and foster each muscle of the body, yet in addition direct the flow of blood, sanitize the lungs, move the mind and accordingly accomplish an agreeable improvement of youngsters character. Various yogic practices are being done by top sportsmen and world champions of many countries as a form of conditioning or relaxation exercises. Problem solving ability is the act of turning new and imaginative ideas into reality. Problem solving ability is characterized by the ability to perceive the world in new ways, to find hidden patterns, to make connections between seemingly unrelated phenomena, and to generate solutions. Problem solving ability involves two processes: thinking, then producing. If you have ideas, but don't act on them, you are imaginative but not creative. Problem solving ability begins with a foundation of knowledge, learning a discipline, and mastering a way of thinking. You learn to be creative by experimenting, exploring, questioning assumptions, using imagination and synthesing information. Learning to be creative is akin to learning a sport. It requires practice to develop the right muscles, and a supportive environment in which to flourish. Problem solving ability is a phenomenon whereby something new and valuable is created (such as an idea, a joke, an artistic or literary work, a painting or musical composition, a solution, an invention etc.). The ideas and concepts so conceived can then manifest themselves in any number of ways, but most often, they become something we can see, hear, smell, touch, or taste.

Memory is the sum totals of what we remember, and gives us the capability to learn and adapt from previous experiences as well as to build relationships. It is the ability to remember past experiences and the power or process of recalling to mind previously learned facts, experiences, impressions, skills and habits. It is the store of things learned and retained from our activity or experience, as evidenced by modification of structure or behavior, or by recall and recognition. Etymologically, the modern English word "memory" comes to us from the Middle English memorie, which in turn comes from the Anglo- French memoire or memorie, and ultimately from the Latinmemoria and memor, meaning "mindful" or "remembering". Memory is concerned with mind. It is one type of strength and it is capacity of one's mind. The learner whose mind is sharp can remember the learnt or taught content. Yogasana can sharpen the capacity, ability and strength of children's mind. Memory is concerned with mind. It is one type of strength and it is capacity of one's mind. The learner whose mind is sharp can remember the learnt or taught content. Yogasana can sharpen the capacity, ability and strength of children's mind. Important memories typically move from short-term memory to long-term memory. The transfer of information to long-term memory for more permanent storage can be happen in several steps. Information can be committed to long-term memory through repetition such as studying for a test or repeatedly taking steps until walking can be performed without thinking or associating it with other previously acquired knowledge, like remembering a new acquaintance.

Problem solving ability is also a consideration, in that information relating to something that you have a keen interest in is more likely to be stored in your long-term memory. That's why someone might be able to recall the stats of a favorite cricket player years after he has retired or where a favorite pair of shoes was purchased. Keeping this point in mind the investigator has selected the topic whether memory and Problem solving ability are affected by yogasana training. It has also been approved fact that a mind can only remain sound if the body is sound. Sound physical and mental health can accelerate the pace of learning and performance in different fields.

STATEMENT OF THE PROBLEM

The purpose of the study was to see the "**Effect of Yoga on Memory and Problem Solving Ability of Players**".

OBJECTIVES

The present study asserts to meet the following objectives

1) To find out the effect of the Yoga on Memory of Players.
2) To find out the effect of the Yoga on Problem Solving Ability of Players.
3) To find out the correlation between Memory and Problem Solving Ability of Players.

HYPOTHESIS OF THE STUDY

On the basis of the knowledge reflected by the available literature, research finding, experts opinion and the scholars own understanding of the problem it was hypothesized that:

1-There will be no significant difference of Yoga on Memory of Players.

- 1. a). There will be no significant difference of Yoga on Remote Memory of Players.
- 1. b). There will be no significant difference of Yoga on Recent Memory of Players.
- 1. c). There will be no significant difference of Yoga on Mental Balance of Players.
- 1. d). There will be no significant difference of Yoga on Attention and Concentration of Players.
- 1. e). There will be no significant difference of Yoga on Delayed Recall of Players.
- 1. f). There will be no significant difference of Yoga on Immediate Recall of Players.
- 1. g). There will be no significant difference of Yoga on Retention for Similar Pairs of Players.
- 1. h). There will be no significant difference of Yoga on Retention for Dissimilar pairs of Players.
- 1. i). There will be no significant difference of Yoga on Visual Retention of Players.

- 1. j). There will be no significant difference of Yoga on Recognition of Players.

2-There will be no significant difference of Yoga on Problem Solving Ability of Players.

3-There will be no significant Correlation between Memory and Problem Solving Ability of Players.

DELIMITATION OF STUDY

Keeping in view the limitations of time and other resources available, the present study was confined to the following delimitation:

- Related research work was delimited to the players of Universities of Haryana (Chaudhary Devi lal University, Sirsa; Chaudhary Ranbir Singh University, Jind; Kurukshetra University, Kurukshetra; Maharishi Dayanand University, Rohtak).
- Related research work was delimited to psychological test PGI Memory Scale developed by Dwarka Pershad (1977) and Problem Solving Ability Test developed by L.N. Dubey (1971).
- Related research work was delimited to the age group between 20 to25 years only.
- The research work was delimited to the 100 players (25 from each university).
- The research work was delimited to Yoga i.e. Asans, Pranayama, Kriya, Surya Namaskar.
- Related research work was delimited to the find out the effect of yogas on Memory (Remote Memory, Recent Memory, Mental Balance, Attention and Concentration, Delayed Recall, Immediate Recall, Retention for Similar pairs, Retention for Dissimilar Pairs, Visual Retention and recognition) and Problem Solving Ability of Players.

LIMITATIONS OF STUDY

The present study was the following limitation.

- All the players of the present study belong to Haryana.
- It was beyond control of the lifestyle and daily routine of players.

- The tool for collecting data was based on a psychological questionnaire.
- The data was based on the thoughts of the responders, which will not be completely free from these individual biases and prejudice.

DEFINITIONS OF THE TERMS USED

Yoga: According to Yoga Sutras: Yoga is the removal of the fluctuations of the mind.

According to Oxford (1990): Yoga - Hindu system of philosophic Meditation and asceticism designed to reunion with the universal spirit.

Memory: According to Dr J. Z. Patel: Memory consists in remembering what has previously been learnt.

Problem Solving Ability: According to Thomas J. D'Zurilla (1995): Problem Solving as a "cognitive–affective–behavioral process through which an individual (or group) attempts to identify, discover, or invent effective means of coping with problems encountered in everyday living".

Asana: According to Joshi (1960): The Static condition and posture of the body, delightfully was called asana.

Pranayam: According to Swami Kuvalayendra (1993): Pranayam to get control over the taking and releasing breath according to desire is called.

SIGNIFICANCE OF THE STUDY

Being the tallest, fastest, or strongest athlete in the world is great, but if a sportsperson lacks mental/cognitive skills, his or her entire performance will suffer. In the past, studies compared the psychological traits of players. Surprisingly, athletes psychological capacity has not been evaluated from a cross-cultural perspective.

In this regard, memory and problem-solving ability were evaluated in the current study since these two variables contain a wide range of psychological and cognitive elements. As a result, the findings of the proposed study will shed light on differences in memory and problem-solving ability among Haryana players, allowing sports psychologists to develop even more effective psycho-cognitive programmes for players while taking into account the impact of cultural diversity on these two variables.

- The study may be helpful to improve the physical and psychological status of individual.
- This study would promote awareness of physical activity and yoga among students, parents and teachers.
- The results of the study may highlight that if yoga training is effective for the selected variables.
- It would provide guidance and new knowledge to the physical education and yoga teachers.
- It shall promote children interest in yogasana.
- The study shall be torch bearer for the future investigators who were interested to find out the prevailing situation in children mental abilities and problem solving abilities.
- Maintaining a good mental health is crucial to live a long healthy life. Good mental health can enhance sportsmanship quality of life, while poor mental health can prevent players from living and enhancing life.

SAMPLE AND TRAINING PROGRAMME

To achieve this purpose of the study, have been selected from the different universities of Haryana i.e. Chaudhary Devi Lal University (CDLU), Sirsa; Chaudhary Ranbir Singh University (CRSU), Jind; Kurukshetra University, Kurukshetra (KUK); Maharshi Dayanand University (MDU), Rohtak. The age group range lies between 20 to 25 years. Furthermore, these one hundred students have been divided equally into 4 groups on a University basis, consisting of 25 students each. Here all groups have gone through common yoga protocol exercise for two hours daily during morning and evening sessions for 6 days per week during a four weeks training programme.

CRITERION MEASURES AND PROCEDURE FOR DATA COLLECTION

The data on Memory was assessed by a memory scale PGI Memory Scale (PGIMS) constructed by D. Pershad and N.N. Wig (1977). It contains 10 sub-test- remote memory, recent memory, mental balance, attention-concentration, delayed recall, immediate recall, retention for dissimilar parts, visual retention and recognition. Subjects were well explained before filling up the questionnaire and each subject was given a pen along with the questionnaire. In case of any doubt regarding the statement the researcher clarified the same to the subjects. Filling up the questionnaire took only 15-20 minutes and it was collected back after being filled up. Scoring PGI Memory Scale contains 10 sub-test remote memory, recent memory, mental balance, attention-concentration, delayed recall, immediate recall, retention for dissimilar parts, visual retention and recognition. After scoring of each sub tests, the scores were added for total score of the full test. The maximum possible score for the full test was 115.

The data collected of Problem Solving Ability was assessed using students' examination problem solving ability tests by L.N. Dubey (1971). This test consists of 20 problems. Each problem has four alternative answers. The duration of this test is 40 minutes. To measure the Problem Solving ability of the subjects, the first test was conducted before the beginning training program. It was administered again after completion of the training program. For the conduct of the test, players were distributed a problem solving ability test. They were asked to mask the correct answer in the test. The total time for the test was 40 minutes. It was instructed to the player that maximum attempts should be made within stipulated 40 minutes time. Scoring each problem has four alternative answers. Out four answers one is correct. If the player writes the correct answer he/she should be given one mark, if the answer is wrong then they get zero marks. The duration of this test is 40 minutes.

EXPERIMENTAL DESIGN

The pre and post test randomized groups design was adopted for this study. All the subjects were divided into four groups each comprising 25 subjects. Each group had students of equal status with respect to age, diet, socio economic conditions. Further, the experimental treatments were also assigned randomly to all experimental groups. All the groups were assigned specific yogic training programmes consisting of Asanas, Pranayamas and Surya Namaskar and Kriya after general warming up. The training was carried out for a total duration of four weeks. The subject voluntarily participated in the study. All the four groups were pre tested as well as post tested on the selected components of psychological areas.

STATISTICAL TECHNIQUES USED

As a statistical measure was carried out using IBM SPSS (Statistical Package for Social Sciences) statistical version 20. All quantitative variables were estimated using measures of central location (mean and median) and measures of dispersion (standard deviation). Normality of data was checked by Skewness and Kurtosis. For normality distributed data, Mean was compared in with respect to One way ANOVA (for more than two groups) and after One way ANOVA significant using Post hoc Least Significant Difference Test (LSD) for multiple comparison. For normality distributed data, Mean was compared pre and post using Dependent t-test. For normality distributed data, Pearson Correlation Method was used for relationship between parameters. All statistical tests were seen at two-tailed levels of significance ($p \leq 0.01$ and $p \leq 0.05$). ANOVA and t-test were used to analyze the data collected from experimental and control group, before and after yoga training of university players through SPSS software.

DISCUSSION OF THE RESULT

On the basis of the statistical analyses of the data, the results were as follows.

There will be no significant difference of yoga on memory of players after study we had rejected the null hypothesis for F-test and can presume that there was a measurably huge distinction in the after effects of the memory trial of the players prior to going to the yoga camp, had a place with various universities of Haryana. A few investigations had featured the mental, for instance, Schaeffer (2002) guaranteed "yoga can forestall memory slips by quieting you and improving your fixation. It can likewise improve your forces of review by expanding dissemination to your mind." Specifically, two rearranged presents are recommended, the open-legged forward bend and threading the needle.

There will be no significant difference of yoga on remote memory of players. After analysis of the study for remote memory test, the t-value was 3.124 with p-value 0.002 which was highly strong to reject the null hypothesis of t-test and conclude that there was highly significant difference in results of remote memory test of the players, before and after attending the yoga camp. Result of this study was almost in line with our study, Shashi (1989) used five intellectual tests (shading abrogation, digit forward, digit in reverse, acknowledgment, and visual maintenance) to contemplate the impacts of yoga over the period of time of a scholastic year for 12 year old members. Results showed enhancement for most tests from the start to the furthest limit of the school year both for a gathering that routinely took an interest in yoga and a gathering that did not accepted.

There will be no significant difference of yoga on recent memory of players of players, the t-value for recent memory test was 6.102 with p-value 0.001 (highly significant), hence we could reject the null hypothesis for t-test and can infer that there was highly significant difference in results of recent memory test of the players, before and after attending the yoga camp. The effect of yogic exercise on the mind is aid to have immediate effects. Kocher (1979) used both meaningful words and nonsense syllables to test immediate (short-term) verbal memory abilities before and after a one-month period of yoga training for college-aged males and females. The results, though incomplete, suggested that yoga did facilitate immediate memory performance more than the absence of yoga, and that the benefit was greater for males than for females.

There will be no significant difference of yoga on mental balance of players. With the t-value of 0.114 and p-value 0.910 for mental balance test, we could not reject the null hypothesis, hence we accept the null hypothesis of t-test for mental balance, and there was no significant difference in the mental balance test of the players for before and after attending the yoga camp. Present study also shows that Yoga has become a very popular recreational activity for many Americans. A relationship between the practice of yoga and benefits related to mental balance and overall wellness is apparent (Schaeffer, 2002).

There will be no significant difference of yoga on attention and concentration of players. Similarly, for attention and concentration test, t-value was 1.481 and p-value was 0.142 which was very weak to reject the null hypothesis, hence we conclude that there was no significant difference in the attention and concentration test of the players, before and after attending the yoga camp. Moreover, changes were seen on attention and concentration level of yoga players after three months of yoga training. These findings were almost in line with the result of this study specifically, inverted yogsa position have been associated with claims of increased memory and attention due to increased blood flow to the brain. For example, Schaeffer (2002) claimed "yoga can prevent memory lapses by claiming you and enhancing your concentration. All mentioned studies found similar results on the attention and concentration of players after yoga trainings. The findings of the study were in agreement with the results of Das (2019), Kallivayalil (2021).

There will be no significant difference of yoga on delayed recall of players. The t-value was 5.173 with p-value of 0.001 which was highly significant; hence we could reject the null hypothesis of t-test and conclude that there was a highly significant difference in the results of the delayed recall test of the players for before and after attending the yoga camp. NK, M., & Telles, S. (2004) the purpose of the study was to find out the effect of Spatial and verbal memory test scores following yoga and fine arts camps for school children. The groups of thirty students equally divided into two groups and aged 11 to 16 years were there. One group attended a yoga camp and the other a fine arts camp. Both groups were assessed on the memory tasks pre and after ten days of their respective interventions. A control group (n= 30) was similarly studied to assess the test–retest effect. At the final assessment the yoga group showed a significant increase of 43% in spatial memory scores (Multivariate analysis, Tukey test), while the fine arts and control groups showed no change. The results suggested that yoga practice, including physical postures, yoga breathing, meditation and guided relaxation improved delayed recall of spatial information.

There will be no significant difference of yoga on immediate recall of players. The t-value was 4.814 and p-value is 0.001which was very strong to reject the null hypothesis of t-test and hence, we could conclude that there was a highly significant difference in the results of the immediate recall test of the players after attending the yoga camp. The effect of yogic exercises on the mind is said to have immediate effects. Kocher (1974) used both meaningful words and nonsense syllables to test immediate (short-term) verbal memory abilities before and after a one-month period of yoga training for college-aged males and females. The results, though incomplete, suggested that yoga did facilitate immediate memory performance more than the absence of yoga, and that the benefit was greater for males than for females.

There will be no significant difference of yoga on retention for similar pairs of players. The t-value was 0.564 with p-value of 0.574 which was very weak to reject the null hypothesis of t-test, hence we accept the null hypothesis, so there was no significant difference in the results of retention for similar pairs test of the players in case of before and after attending the yoga camp Sahasi (1989) utilized five cognitive tests (color cancellation, digit forward, digit backward, recognition, and visual retention) to study the effects of yoga over the time span of an academic year for 12 year old participants. Results showed improvement on most tests from the beginning to the end of the school year both for a group that regularly participated in yoga and a group that did not.

There will be no significant difference of yoga on retention for dissimilar pairs of players. The t-value was 18.482 with p-value of 0.001 which was very strong to reject the null hypothesis of t-test, hence we reject the null hypothesis, and so there was highly significant difference in the results of retention for dissimilar pair's test of the players, in case of before and after attending the yoga camp. Kioumourtzoglou et al. (1998) "aim of this study to assess cognitive, perceptual and motor skill ability in elite Basketball players". Thirteen (n-13) men of elite male national team of Basketball players were selected as a sample for laboratory study aged lies between 22 to 23 years and fifteen men of same age (physical education class) were selected to assess difference in their scores on cognitive skill (memory-retention, memory grouping analytics ability), perceptual skill (speed of perception, prediction ,selective attention, response selection and motor skills (dynamic balance, whole body coordination, wrist - finger dexterity, rhythmic ability). The result shows that those who are elite Basketball players score better on memory-retention, selective attention, and on prediction measures than the control group.

There will be no significant difference of yoga on visual retention of players. The t-value of 2.091 with p-value 0.039 for visual retention test indicates the significant p-value, hence we could reject the null hypothesis for t-test and conclude that there was a significant difference in the visual retention. It was evident from the above finding that test of the players Cowen and Adams (2005) have evaluated the impact of six weeks of either ashtanga yoga or hatha yoga classes. Significant improvements in follow-up were observed in all participants in diastolic blood pressure, upper body and stem muscle strength and endurance, flexibility, visual stress, and health perception. Progress given by each group compared to basic tests. The group of astanga yoga has lowered diastolic blood pressure and visual acuity, and increased body and stem muscle strength and endurance, flexibility, and a sense of well-being. The development of the hatha yoga group was only important for trunk muscle strength and endurance and flexibility. The findings suggest that the benefits of practicing yoga vary in style.

There will be no significant difference of yoga on recognition of players for recognition test, with t-value 1.288 and p-value 0.201 we could not reject the null hypothesis; hence we accept the null hypothesis that there was a non-significant difference in the recognition test of the players for before and after attending the yoga camp. Raingruber (2007) the outcomes of the self-care classes described by nurses include: (a) awareness of warmth, tingling, and relaxation, (b) awareness of improved problem-solving ability, and (c) recognition of increased ability to focus on patient needs. Hospitals willing to invest in nursing care options can expect patient and work-related benefits. The scientific studies related Kioumourtzoglou et al (1998) aim of this study to assess cognitive, perceptual and motor skill ability in elite Basketball players. Thirteen (n-13) men of elite male national team of Basketball players were selected as a sample for laboratory study aged lies between 22 to 23 years and fifteen men of same age (physical education class) were selected to assess difference in their scores on cognitive skill (memory-retention, memory grouping analytics ability), perceptual skill (speed of perception, prediction ,selective attention, response selection and motor skills (dynamic balance, whole body coordination, wrist - finger dexterity, rhythmic ability). The result shows that those who are elite Basketball players score better on memory-retention, selective attention, and on prediction measures than the control group. NK, M., & Telles, S. (2004) the purpose of the study was to find out the effect of Spatial and verbal memory test scores following yoga and fine arts camps for school children. The groups of thirty students equally divided into two groups and aged 11 to 16 years were there. One group attended a yoga camp and the other a fine arts camp. Both groups were assessed on the memory tasks pre and after ten days of their respective interventions. A control group (n= 30) was similarly studied to assess the test–retest effect. At the final assessment the yoga group showed a significant increase of 43% in spatial memory scores (Multivariate analysis, Tukey test), while the fine arts and control groups showed no change. The results suggested that yoga practice, including physical postures, yoga breathing, and meditation and guided relaxation improved delayed recall of spatial information.

There will be no significant difference of yoga on problem solving ability of players. We could reject the null hypothesis for F-test and can conclude that there was a statistically significant difference in the results of the problem-solving ability test of the players before attending the yoga camp, belong to different universities of

Haryana. Fatin Abdullah et al. (2005) investigated physics problem solving skills of secondary students in relation to ethnicity. Five students achieving the highest scores on both the Physics Problems Solving Ability Test (PPSAT) and the Metacognitive Skills Questionnaire (MSQ) were selected to be reassessed using the qualitative techniques. The qualitative techniques are thinking aloud protocol, interviews and analysis of the paper & pencil test by the students. The cross tabulation and triangulation techniques were implied and the results were later being compared with the past researches found in the literature. This study was conducted in Malaysia. It was found that ethnicity has a significant effect on the problem solving ability of secondary students. It was observed that Chinese students have more magnitude of problem solving skills as compared to Malay students but no significant difference was observed in problem solving skills of Indian and Chinese as well as Indian and Malay students. The results showed a partial effect of ethnicity on problem solving skills of secondary students.

There will be no significant correlation between memory and problem-solving ability of players. Likewise, result of PGI memory scale test of players was positively correlated with results of the problem-solving ability test with correlation coefficient of 0.096, but the correlation was non-significant as the p-values was greater than 0.05. Before and after attending the yoga camp, hence we could not reject the Hypothesis 3. Therefore, we accept the H03 hypothesis, so there was no significant correlation between the memory and problem-solving ability of players. It was evident from the above finding that Shahbazi (2018) studied the effect of problem solving skill training on emotional intelligence of nursing students. Heidari (2016) studied the effect of problem solving training on decision –making skill and critical thinking in emergency medical personnel.

CPSIA information can be obtained
at www.ICGtesting.com
Printed in the USA
LVHW050811090123
736650LV00011BA/842